Walking The Crooked Path

Corey King

ISBN: **1500228427**
ISBN-13: **978-1500228422**

ACKNOWLEDGEMENTS

Many people have walked with me, supported me, encouraged me, chastised me, and made my journey richer and more rewarding. I wish I could thank them all, but then the acknowledgements would be longer than the book. However, some I must acknowledge individually.

To my friends in the PD advocacy community—thank you for being there for me, and allowing me to be there for you.

To Ronnie, my friend and colleague, and my last in a long string of bosses—you are a great leader, manager, and engineer, and you're a wise and compassionate man completely dedicated to doing what's right. Thank you.

To Larry—thank you for asking your question, and for sticking with me while I answered it. Thanks for your constant, unflagging support, even when I didn't know it was there. And thanks for introducing me to the guys.

To Ken—I've walked the path with you my entire life, and although you're a phenomenal brother who's looked out for me and protected me, you're an even better friend and traveling companion. I hope the path before us is as long as we both want it to be. I love you, brah.

To Gene—of all the unexpected joys in my life, knowing you may be the greatest. You're my friend, my mentor, my confidante, and my shootin' buddy. More importantly, in you I see both a father and The Father. Thank you, my friend. I love you.

To Jeanette—even though I might have been a little rough around the edges as your first son-in-law, you accepted me, loved me, supported me during the most difficult parts of my journey, and treated me as a son. I'm grateful for your kindness and example, and I love you.

To my children—every father wants his children to be better than he was. Your path is still largely unwalked, but in different ways I see in both of you the things that I've always wanted to be. I'm so proud of you both, and I love you.

And to my beloved wife Amy—our path together has been exceedingly crooked at times, but we've always walked together. Even when you've been angry enough with me to cheerfully strangle me, you've always been there. I regret the times I've taken it for granted, and the times I have lost sight of the important and been distracted by the urgent. The path ahead of me will be difficult, but with you beside me I can do anything. And when I can't, I know you can. *Tu es ma meilleure amie et ma joie de vivre, et je t'aime de tout mon coeur.*

Love builds up the broken wall, and straightens the crooked path…
- *Maya Angelou*

So live your life that the fear of death can never enter your heart…
- *Chief Tecumseh*

I believe; help my unbelief…
- *Mark 9:24*

I'VE GOT WHAT?

I squirmed on the cold plastic chair in the doctor's examining room and thumbed through a limp copy of Texas Monthly Magazine, muttering to myself. I was already late for a meeting and I didn't have time for this nonsense. There was nothing wrong with me that I couldn't explain; sure, my hands and arms were stiff and sore, and occasionally didn't work quite the way I told them to, but I was sure the pain and stiffness were the result of creeping middle age and overexertion. I had taught a group of scuba students just a few days before, and I was always a little tired and sore after a class.

I hummed tunelessly along with a Muzak version of Elton John's "Rocket Man," and resisted the impulse to rummage through the drawers looking for rubber gloves to make balloon animals. I had just learned that the doctor was out, and my irritation level was climbing. I grumbled a string of complaints, "Waste of time... nothing really wrong with me... I need to get back to work... she always thinks she knows better than me... this song sucks... just overdid it in class last week... doctor's not even here today... wonder what she'll think of THAT... don't even have any good magazines..."

For more than ten years, the ache and stiffness in my left shoulder, elbow, and wrist had been a constant, unwelcome companion. My left hand and fingers were clumsy, I unconsciously carried my left arm curled against my chest, and I had developed a slight limp. Friends and colleagues asked, "What's with your arm? Why are you limping? You look stiff—what's wrong?"

I dismissed the questions with a variety of plausible explanations: weekend tree-trimming, old skiing injuries, ill-fitting shoes, overexertion in scuba classes. The symptoms had grown over more than a decade, so slowly that I didn't notice. Irritated and perplexed, I stiff-armed the well-intentioned concerns. After all, who knew better than me if something serious was wrong? I was always the smartest guy in the room: no one, especially doctors who had never met me before, could tell me something about myself that I didn't know first.

My wife Amy is blessed with many wonderful qualities, but patience and tact aren't always at the top of the list. Perhaps it's just the effect I have on her. She could also see physical changes in me, but she was as much a victim of the "boiling frog" phenomenon as I was—the changes were so gradual that she wasn't consciously aware of them either. She had an intuition that something serious was amiss, though, and it scared her. Fear usually manifests as anger with her, and that fear coupled with her self-described "Texas redneck" approach to problem solving resulted in colorful conversations.

"My arms don't move right. Look at this." I demonstrated moving my right arm and hand, making normal iron-pumping movements and clenching my fist rapidly.

"Yeah? So?"

"Well, look what happens with my left arm." I repeated the demonstration, and instead of rapid, smooth motion, my left hand and arm quivered spastically, jerked, and thrashed like a fish trying to throw a hook.

"You're doing that on purpose."

"I swear I'm not," I assured her.

"That's pretty messed up, hon. Why don't you go see a doctor?"

"Oh, I don't have time. Besides, they don't know anything."

"You always go in and tell them what's wrong, Ignatz. Why don't you try telling them what hurts then let them decide what's wrong?"

I choose to believe that "Ignatz" means "intelligent and noble love of my life" in a language that I don't speak.

I said, "Okay, but not next week. I'm going to DC next week, and then I've got a meeting with a client, and then…"

She rolled her eyes at me and walked away, and we tabled the subject until the next time I felt the need to demonstrate the right-left disparity.

Visiting the doctor was just below being water boarded on my list of favorite things, so several years passed before I made an appointment for a checkup. While I procrastinated, new physical difficulties emerged. The buttons on my shirt cuffs and collars inexplicably grew larger; pushing them through the buttonholes became a daily morning struggle. My neckties and shoelaces joined the rebellion, and resentfully resisted all my efforts to bend them into pleasing and useful shapes. Through years of repetition, I had honed my morning ritual to maximize sleep time: twenty-three minutes from alarm to key-in-ignition, backing out of the garage. As that time stretched from thirty minutes, to forty-five, to over an hour, I developed an uncomfortable suspicion that I was facing something more serious than simple laziness and middle-aged malaise.

I finally made an appointment for an annual physical. "Annual" was an exaggeration, since my last was over five years before. The doctor had some catching up to do. She proceeded with a detailed medical history, poked, prodded, took samples of various fluids, encouraged me to cough, and attached me to machines that plumbed my body's secrets.

As the exam came to an end, I mentioned, "Oh, I've been having problems with my left hand and arm—they hurt and feel stiff, and my hand shakes sometimes and it doesn't move right." I demonstrated.

The doctor agreed, although she didn't call me "Ignatz"—we only know each other casually, and I'm clearly not the love of her life. "Well, yes—that probably shouldn't happen. Have you hurt your arm recently?"

We discussed several possibilities, including arthritis and joint problems from a variety of old football, baseball, skiing, and beer pong injuries. She talked about the wide-ranging effects of neck and shoulder damage, referred me to an orthopedic surgeon, and sent me on my way.

I saw orthopedic surgeons for my neck, shoulder, elbow, and hand, received multiple cortisone injections, had a series of MRIs and x-rays, and finally saw a neurologist for an electromyogram. This delightful procedure involves electricity and needles, and when the neurologist told me what he planned to do, I thought he was joking. He wasn't.

"So, you're really going to stick needles in my hand and arm, hook them up to a generator, and run current through them?" I asked.

"Well, it's slightly more technically sophisticated than that, but essentially, yes."

"And, by doing this, you hope to learn… what?"

"That's a little complex for the layman to understand, but rest assured, there's a purpose."

I imagine Jack the Ripper told his victims something similar, but I kept my mouth shut, hoping not to goad the doctor into higher voltage levels than strictly necessary. I thought I heard screams coming from his other examining rooms (no doubt in a nearby dungeon), but I'm sure my imagination was just in overdrive.

He inserted the needles and said, "Now, hold still." He cranked up the juice.

"I thought I told you to hold still; you're corrupting the data."

I was comforted to know he was actually collecting data and not engaging in some bizarre recreational activity, so I gritted my teeth, manfully didn't suggest that we switch places so he could be still and I could run the generator, and tried to stop my involuntary shaking. I couldn't, and both my anxiety level and his grumbling increased. After an eternity of jolts and tickles, he removed the needles and chased me out of his office, muttering about simple procedures and uncooperative patients.

The EMG indicated minor nerve problems in my elbow. I discussed the results with one of a series of orthopedic surgeons, and asked what I should do next. He told me he thought my symptoms would improve with elbow surgery to reduce nerve irritation and pressure. Feeling a little irritated myself, I asked, "Will surgery help with the shaking and stiffness, too?"

"Well, I really don't know what's causing that, but I think you should consider the surgery anyway," he said.

"So, you're not sure what's causing the symptoms, but surgery is the answer?"

Giving me a look that indicated that he, too, considered me to be an uncooperative patient, he said, "We could always try another cortisone injection." I suspected that his knife and needle were solutions in search of a problem I didn't have, so I thanked him and said I'd consider his advice. He was as glad to see me go as I was.

On a short vacation a few months later, as Amy and I walked together through Manhattan, I noticed she was avoiding walking on my right side.

"You keep whacking me with that darn college ring of yours when I'm on your right. You bruise me less when I'm on your left. You don't swing your left arm."

"Really? How long's that been going on?"

"Oh, I never really thought about it. Maybe ten or fifteen years—a long time," she replied. I hadn't noticed, but I realized she was right: my left arm didn't swing when I walked.

Over the next few months I noticed other anomalies. On a business trip to Washington DC in the winter of 2008, as a colleague and I walked back to our hotel after dinner, I had trouble keeping up with her. She said, "You've been dragging around all day, and you look stiff and you're limping. What's up?"

I was walking with a slow, uneven gait and dragging my left leg slightly. My left leg and hip, apparently taking lessons from my left arm and shoulder, were stiff and sore. My colleague was recovering from hip replacement surgery, but she had to wait for me to catch up with her a dozen times on the walk from dinner back to the hotel.

The collection of physical problems began to form a pattern, but I didn't see it. I enthusiastically explained away each anomaly—the shoulder pain was from a skiing injury, the neck stiffness was from a foolish, drunken encounter with the shallow bottom of Lake Austin that nearly left me paralyzed, the tingling and clumsiness in my left hand were due to nerve damage from either my neck or shoulder, the elbow pain was from carrying scuba tanks in diving classes, the leg pain was from muscle strain at the gym, or maybe from the new shoes that didn't quite fit. I always had an answer, and it was always wrong.

Amy finally ran completely out of patience and made an appointment with a specialist in internal medicine. "Just go," she told me. "Keep your mouth shut and answer his questions, and let him do his job."

I bit back a snarky comment about the difficulty of both answering his questions and keeping my mouth shut. I surrendered to the inevitable, but I thought, "I'll go, but he's not going to tell me anything I don't already know."

I knew something was wrong. Cancer, strokes, high blood pressure, and diabetes, which were all a part of my genetic background, explained some of the symptoms, but nothing I knew explained them all. My mother and father had both died only a few years before, and between their two medical histories I was potentially at risk for almost everything. I figured I had all the data I needed and that this was a puzzle I could solve. After all, why trust the doctors? They had repeatedly been wrong, and I was convinced I could do at least as well at diagnosis as they could.

The Muzak was now playing a watered-down, almost unrecognizable version of a Metallica song, and as I considered sneaking out the back door and coming back in a couple of years, the door opened and a nurse entered, bringing with her a whirlwind of activity. She was professional and competent, and I felt a little ashamed of myself. I still believed I was the smartest guy in the room, but only because I was the only guy in the room.

She began by taking a detailed medical history, and then introduced me to the neurological test I would later know as the "hokey-pokey exam." Finger taps, toe taps, fist clenching, heel stomping, put your left leg in, take your left leg out... it would have been difficult under the best of circumstances, and to my surprise, I performed poorly on many parts of the exam. I could tap my right index finger and thumb together at a rapid, regular pace, but my left hand lagged behind, and the same was true of any test that required coordinated movement between my left and right side.

"My wife claims I can't dance, either—maybe I have an excuse," I joked. The nurse glanced at me and continued the exam.

"There are several tests we can't do here that I'd like to order for you," she said. She suggested multiple blood tests and a brain scan, commenting, "With your symptoms, a brain tumor is always a possibility and needs to be ruled out." Brain tumor? Brain tumor?? Elbow surgery looked good by comparison—let's go back to that, I thought.

She finished the exam and left me alone again in the examination room while she made appointments for what seemed like several thousand additional tests, including a brain MRI. I finally left the office with a handful of orders and instructions to come back with the results.

In addition to donating several gallons of blood and urine to the testing gods, I spent an hour stuffed inside a cramped, noisy MRI machine, listening to a loud hammering sound and trying not to move. I was only partially successful; the MRI technician repeatedly called out to me by microphone from the control booth, "You're moving—if you don't stop, we'll have to repeat the test." I felt like a recalcitrant five-year-old being scolded for wiggling in church.

The torture finally ceased, and I collected my images and x-rays. The internist had arranged an appointment with a neurologist to discuss the imaging tests, and so in the summer of 2009, almost fifteen years after I first noticed a persistent ache in my left arm, I met with the neurologist.

It was the same neurologist who had performed my medieval torture test. I verified that electrified needles weren't on the schedule, and he looked at my brain images and pronounced them unremarkable.

I bristled. I liked my brain and it had served me well; I was offended that he didn't see evidence that it was a remarkable organ. In a tone that reminded me he hadn't forgotten my tendency to be uncooperative, he told me that to a doctor, "unremarkable" means, "I don't see anything here that's going to kill you," rather than, "what a boring, ordinary brain." He took a detailed medical history and then performed a much more comprehensive hokey-pokey exam. He finally completed his evaluation. We sat down, and he proceeded to change my life forever.

"I'm sorry, but your symptoms, tests, and medical history indicate Parkinsonism, most likely idiopathic Parkinson's disease. We'll need to do more tests, but I'm confident that's what you have."

I was shocked and almost incoherent. Through the fog of white noise in my mind, I tried to form reasonable thoughts and questions, but my first response was not the most complex thought I've ever had.

"Naaaah, can't be." I raised several objections, and the doctor patiently addressed each of them.

"But I'm too young for Parkinson's."

"Parkinson's affects people of all ages, although it's more common after age sixty. You probably have something called young-onset PD, but as I said, we'll need to do more testing to be sure," he replied.

"It's only on one side."

"That's not at all unusual. As a matter of fact, that's how it usually starts."

"I don't shake all that much. Isn't Parkinson's disease mostly about tremors?"

"The primary symptom of PD is often a rest tremor, but it doesn't have to be, especially in young-onset patients," he replied.

For the next fifteen minutes, I continued to search for the question that would undermine his diagnosis, and he continued to answer them all. He then told me he wanted to start me on a Parkinson's medication. If my symptoms improved, it would reinforce his diagnosis.

The long delay and uncertainty between my initial noticeable symptoms and an accurate diagnosis were frustrating but not unusual. PD can be difficult to diagnose, especially in younger people. The symptoms are subtle and gradual, and can have many causes. Doctors are taught to think of the most common causes first, and to leave the more exotic conclusions until the obvious and mundane has been ruled out. "When you hear hoof beats, think horses and not zebras," they say.

PD is a zebra, and is unusual enough in a younger person that it's often not considered until other diagnoses prove to be wrong. That's partially why my diagnosis was so difficult. My own insistence that I knew more than the entire medical establishment complicated the process, though, and injected additional delay and confusion.

My crooked path to the knowledge that I am a person with Parkinson's—or PWP—was only the first part of a longer journey. Along the way, I'm learning to cope not only with the physical and mental symptoms of an incurable, degenerative neurological disease, but also with radical changes in self-perception and outlook. PD changes everything; it has forced me to reexamine my identity, my most basic beliefs, and my purpose in living. It has changed my relationships with people I love, led me to reconsider my understanding of trust and control, and challenged everything I thought was true.

I'm also learning that even when my fellow travelers disappear and the path looks deserted, I'm still not alone. Parkinson's disease will eventually take everything, but in return it's giving me a surprising faith that I didn't expect and had actively resisted for my entire life. PD stripped away my pretensions and forced me to confront questions I thought I had answered long ago and wounds I thought were long healed.

There's an old Yiddish saying that I've always liked: "Man plans, and God laughs." Perhaps the idea is better stated in Proverbs 16:9, though: "In their hearts men plan their course, but the Lord establishes their steps." For most of my life, I've been convinced that I was in charge of my destination and that I chose the steps I took. I've come to realize that I've been wrong. God has apparently been gently amused at my presumption, and He has my attention now.

INITIATION

One of my first memories is of a bright light suspended above me. I learned later, as part of the set of stories I've come to call our "family mythology," that the light was a chandelier shaped like a wagon wheel hanging above the breakfast table in our house in south Dallas. It fascinated me, and I reached for the light from my high chair during meals with my parents, my big sister, and two older brothers gathered around the table. According to family mythology, the light was also the source of my first words—as I reached for the sparkling brightness with rapt attention, they repeated, "That's a light, Corey; light. Can you say 'light'?" They were overjoyed when I responded obediently, "ligh…," and they provided the proper correction.

"No, it's 'light'. Say 'light'."

I don't remember being irritated at the correction, but my second word was "…ighT," as if to say, "I GET it. Don't bother me."

I am the youngest in my family by six years, and family mythology also states that I was "the surprise." I took that to mean that I was unplanned, and I hoped that it was the, "Oh, look, we just won the lottery" type of surprise, rather than the "Oh, look, the dog found a dead muskrat and brought it home" type. The mythology remains silent on this subject.

I was a serious and thoughtful child, and my parents jokingly told me that I was the old man in the family. When my brothers and sister were joking, cutting up, or being loud and boisterous in the car, my parents rarely had to discipline them when I was there. Mimicking the words and tone I had heard, I scolded, "Behave, you kids," in a severe voice.

I earned the nickname "Eeyore," after the donkey in the Winnie the Pooh books that took a dismal view of every situation, expecting to be the butt of all jokes. I didn't see the humor; it was obvious that Eeyore had a clear view and common-sense approach. I wanted to be Christopher Robin, but Eeyore was my kind of guy.

My family told me that I was adopted (nothing wrong with being adopted—I'm not, but have wished occasionally since then that I had been), that I was overweight (my father's nickname for me for years was Tosca Fats—I was built like a greyhound, but that's what made it funny, get it?) and that I was Chinese (since every fourth child born in the world is Chinese, and I was the fourth child in our family). It was all done in good fun, of course, and perhaps with the underlying goal of shaking me out of my serious attitude. I think it worked—now an adult, I think many things are funny that I suspect are actually not.

My sister Kathy doted on me, and was my second mother. She read to me from Winnie the Pooh, told me stories of Little Suzy the squirrel and the toy soldiers who protected her, and introduced me to the mysteries of "One Fish, Two Fish" and "Go, Dogs, Go." She loved the "Peanuts" comic strip, especially Snoopy, and for some unfathomable reason she also liked folk music. I barely survived exposure to The Brothers Four and The Kingston Trio, but I loved reading with her.

The younger of my two brothers, Ken, looked after me and made me laugh. He was my hero. He could do everything I wanted to do, everyone liked him, and he wasn't embarrassed to have me tag along. Over the years, Ken taught me to throw a baseball, climb a tree, tell a joke, talk to girls, and a few other things I might have been better off not learning. I idolized Ken; although Kathy was my second mother, Ken was and will always be my big brother.

My oldest brother, Marc, was a cipher to me. He was quiet and reserved, and his room smelled like English Leather aftershave. He was an Eagle Scout and he liked building airplanes; the balsa wood and tissue paper creations that adorned his room were fascinating, and looked hopelessly complex. I always hoped he would teach me how to cut and glue the tiny wooden parts to make a wing or fuselage, or show me how to fly, but he didn't have much patience for a little brother with too many questions and clumsy fingers. To complicate matters, the fluid that he used to tighten and stiffen the tissue paper on his planes was called "dope." I had heard repeatedly about the dangers of doing dope, so I figured I would be better off avoiding Marc's airplanes, at least until I was older.

I was six. I loved school, had friends, had a crush on the little girl three houses away, and looked forward to the Griff's hamburger my mother bought for me almost every day after half-day kindergarten. My grandfather, whom I called Pappy, took me for haircuts, which were always followed by toys at the Ben Franklin five-and-dime store and ice cream. My favorite was the peppermint stick ice cream at the Polar Bear ice cream shop down the street, and I had the shortest hair of any kid in school; if I could have gotten a haircut every day, I would have been happy. I felt safe and slept soundly at night, and my occasional nightmares faded unremembered with the light of day.

When I was seven, we moved suddenly from Dallas to Washington, DC. I didn't know why we moved, I only knew that everything familiar and comforting in my life had disappeared. My memories of the six months surrounding the move are mostly of whispered conversations that I wasn't supposed to hear. I remember that we moved in the fall after I started first grade. I don't remember much about the previous summer, other than the morning that I learned Marc was in the hospital.

Marc was ten years older, we were not close, and I was slightly afraid of him. He was still my brother, though, and I was upset that he was in the hospital. I was equally upset that no one would tell me why. My father was a policeman, and I knew from other whispered conversations that nothing good comes from sudden visits to the hospital in the middle of the night.

Marc remained in the hospital for several weeks and I was not allowed to visit. In Texas during the 1960s, young children were not welcome during hospital visiting hours, so I moped in the lobby with a succession of relatives—my sister, my mother, my grandmother. I knew something terrible had happened, and my imagination filled in the gaps.

I decided that a monster had attacked Marc. No one wanted me to know, I reasoned, because if the monster knew you were thinking about him, he would come for you, too. I resolved to try very hard not to think about the monster, and thus keep myself safe.

Don't think about a penguin. It's impossible—making a conscious effort to avoid a particular thought practically guarantees failure. Day and night during Marc's hospital stay, I imagined what he looked like, what the monster had done to him, and where the monster was right now. I sweated and shivered in fear, convinced the monster knew I was thinking about him, and I lay awake at night, listening. I knew the monster had taken Marc at night, because he was there when I went to bed and was gone before breakfast. So, I waited. I was dreadfully sure I would be next.

Marc finally came home and confirmed my suspicions. He had been badly injured and walked with silver crutches that wrapped around his forearms and made a disturbing clicking sound. He seemed injured in other ways, too—he seemed not only quiet and reserved, but also angry and withdrawn, and he rarely spoke to me. I grew more afraid, not just of him but of what I imagined had happened to him. I wanted to ask, but even then I recognized the scent of danger in the air—it was a familiar odor in our house. Some subjects were off limits.

Eventually, the monster faded from my conscious thoughts and was replaced with the excitement and anticipation of my first days in "big school." I settled into a first-grade routine of "Tip and Mitten," timed multiplication tests, and civil defense drills. I'm part of the last generation to learn to duck and cover in school, and I vividly remember the teacher blowing her whistle and commanding us to climb under our desks with our backs to the window. I had no idea why we were huddled on the floor, although I knew it had something to do with "the Soviet Union." I had no idea what the Soviet Union was, but I didn't worry excessively. I did wonder why I was safer from it under my desk, though.

I forgot about the monster until the day I came home from school to learn that we were moving. No explanations—I was only a child and wasn't entitled to them. My fears rushed back. The monster had found us again and we were moving to get away, I thought.

It seemed that one moment I was in my familiar bed in Dallas, and the next I was in a new house, in a new school, with teachers I didn't know, surrounded by people I didn't recognize. Kathy was away at college, and amidst the turmoil of the move and my unfamiliar surroundings, my dreadful sense of the monster's presence returned. This time, however, I was confused. Had the monster attacked Marc, or was Marc actually the monster? Through my childish eyes, he even looked like the monster I feared.

Our new house in suburban Maryland was much larger, with empty rooms and hardwood floors. It creaked and echoed. As I lay awake at night, listening to the echoes, I imagined that I could hear the monster moving from room to room.

"Click click, thump, click click, thump, click click, thump…" I knew what I heard was Marc walking upstairs on his crutches, but I imagined the monster was searching the house for me. Maybe those clicking claws and stubby monster feet, thumping down the hall, were coming for me right now.

I huddled in bed as fear and dread trampled through my chest on stubby feet, and in reaction to the stress and anxiety that was common for me over the next ten years, I vomited. The pattern repeated night after night for months. I learned to do my own laundry by washing sheets in the middle of the night so my parents wouldn't know.

They knew, of course. I remember listening through the bedroom wall as my father muttered to my mother, "He does this every night. Can't you keep him quiet?" They both knew. I sometimes wonder if they might even have been proud of me for trying to hide the truth, as if I had learned the family way: "Keep it to yourself; tough it out; no one needs to know our business."

I never knew, and still don't know, the details of Marc's accident. The incident is a taboo subject in the family, not even addressed by the family mythology. Marc won't talk about it even now, at least to me; our relationship is almost non-existent. Over the years, I've pieced together some of the details, attempting to understand—not out of curiosity, but to help fill a hole in my own history and explain a family sickness that still goes uncured. Amidst the rumors, guesses, and speculations now almost fifty years old, the only facts I have found were in a very short article from the Dallas Morning News, dated Tuesday, May 6, 1969, buried in Section D, under Local News:

11

"OFFICER'S SON SHOT IN BACK – The 16-year-old son of a high-ranking Dallas police officer remained in satisfactory condition at Baylor Hospital after he was shot in the back early Sunday morning in a neighbor's home. Police said he was shot once in the lower left back as he tried to flee the home of Bob C. Tinsley, 2233 Tosca Lane, about 2 a.m. Sunday. Tinsley told officers he was awakened by the screams of his wife who told him there was a prowler in their bedroom. Tinsley said the prowler jumped up and ran from the bedroom and into the kitchen. Tinsley chased him, stopping at a closet to get a .22 caliber pistol. He ordered the boy to freeze at the back door, and then fired one shot which hit the youth and a second which struck the door. Police took affidavits from Tinsley and his wife and talked with the boy, a Kimball High School student. Charges were pending a full investigation, police said."

There was no follow-up story, no mention of charges, and no reference to my father anywhere. He was then an assistant chief in the Dallas Police Department, a front-runner to be selected as chief, and Mr. Tinsley, our next-door neighbor, called him first that night. It was my father who found Marc unconscious on the driveway.

I don't know what happened next, but another assistant chief was selected to be chief, my father resigned from the department, and we moved less than six months later. The Dallas Police Department denies having records of the shooting, and it's not clear that there was ever any further investigation. The incident simply evaporated, leaving behind my brother's physical and emotional scars and an unhealed family trauma that continues to fracture us.

My brother was not the monster in the house, nor is his story mine to tell. He was as much of a victim of the real monster as I was. The real monster was secrecy. As I washed sheets in the middle of the night and finally learned to sleep on the bathroom floor when I knew I was going to have a bad night, I learned: when bad things happen, keep quiet.

I had ample opportunity to practice this simple lesson for the next twenty years. I didn't challenge the monster until my own son was born and I could no longer keep a secret I had hidden for almost my entire life. The first person I told was Amy, and she reacted in a way I found familiar—she threw up.

My father, by all appearances a good father, husband, and public servant, molested me repeatedly as a child and young adolescent. I never understood what motivated him, and when I confronted him several years before he died, he couldn't give me any insights. His only interest was in keeping the secret, even after it was out in the open between us—his reaction was to tell me that he didn't think it was necessary for my mother to know about it. For her protection, you see—what use would there be in hurting her?

With Amy's encouragement, I paid him a visit in late 1998 in the retirement community where he lived with my mother in Dallas. I invited him to go for a drive and told him I didn't mind driving. I took his car keys and drove with him for hours through Dallas streets and highways. With him as a literally captive audience, I began asking questions. He handled them all as skillfully as a lifetime in law enforcement, public administration, and executive management could allow. Interrogation was nothing new to him—he had had years of experience before I was even born, and he had nothing to fear from me.

We drove for over four hours. I wanted to see him break. I bludgeoned him with my memories of the things he had done, with his corruption of a relationship that should be sacrosanct. I told him I thought his entire life was a lie, and that nothing he had ever done would matter unless he made this right. I said I didn't trust him around my children, and that was why Amy and I didn't leave them alone with him. I described how it felt to grow up thinking he might kill me someday to keep the secret; if he could do those things to his own son, where were the boundaries? Were there any boundaries at all? I thought I needed him to feel the fear, revulsion, shame, guilt, and confusion he had created in me.

He took it all in stride. He was calm, unperturbed, and as smooth as silk. He might have been screaming on the inside, but he never let it show, and he never expressed regret or asked for forgiveness. I am sure I will never see such a display of misguided, misapplied strength of will again in my life. He died never having raised the subject with me again.

His abuse had two major impacts on my development and outlook. First, I became unable to trust, especially authority figures who claimed to be righteous and virtuous. Father figures, whether in the form of coaches, mentors, military commanders, bosses, or God—the ultimate father figure—were not reliable. I unconsciously and repeatedly searched for a replacement father to trust, and was repeatedly disappointed.

I was also firmly convinced that the abuse was my fault, and that if I had only been stronger, braver, more observant, or more in control, I could have avoided it or stopped it. My father had practiced the application of force and intimidation for his entire adult life, and he was a master at management of people and events, but I still thought I should have stopped him. I became convinced that I was weak and powerless, and my father exploited those feelings as part of the pattern of abuse. Many of my life choices and attitudes can be traced back to my response to my father's abuse.

We all have dark spots on our histories and challenges to overcome. Worse things happen to children at the hands of trusted relatives every day, and my experiences are no excuse for curling up and dying. It's only one of the threads in the tapestry of my life. Like having PD, I would have never wished for it, and I would be heartily grateful if it had never happened, but it eventually helped me to develop the ability to live with adversity, and it led me to believe that I can endure anything.

Even as I write this, though, a voice whispers at the back of my mind, "What are you doing? No one needs to know—you're just embarrassing yourself and everyone else. This is family business—keep your mouth shut."

Throughout my life, this voice has been an overbearing taskmaster, telling me to ignore the truth, hide weakness and failure, and keep family business to myself. Couched in noble terms such as "strong and silent" and "keeping my own counsel," the voice kept me from exposing a family sickness that could have harmed my own children, acknowledging a physical limitation that nearly cost me my life, and coming to terms with Parkinson's disease earlier. The voice once sounded like my father's, but now it's mine. It still whispers, but I've learned not to listen.

INFORMATION AND BELIEF

I left the neurologist's office clutching my bag of medication samples, thinking, "Well. Parkinson's disease. Maybe that's not so bad. Michael J. Fox has Parkinson's, and he's about as cool as they come. And if I only have to take one of these pills a day, I can do that. Yeah—Parkinson's; at least it's not a brain tumor." For a moment, I was relieved to have a label for my collection of physical problems.

Amy was traveling in Africa, so I had time to research and develop a plan to manage the challenge. One little white pill per day and some minor lifestyle changes; no problem, I figured. I'd accomplished harder tasks.

My sense of relief lasted until I sat down in front of my computer. I mentally flipped a coin and settled on Wikipedia, typed in "Parkinson's disease," and started reading.

I read for hours, scarcely believing what I learned. I finally pushed back after ten hours with a myriad of new terms and concepts buzzing in my head and a growing sense of unreality. How could this be? What had I done wrong? I was sure there was a mistake. Parkinson's disease was serious, and except for minor illnesses and middle age, I was healthy. This couldn't be true.

The neurologist instructed me to take the medication he had given me for six weeks. He'd then evaluate the results. Simple and easy, I thought, and definitely will prove I don't have PD.

I swallowed the first pill with a mix of trepidation and anticipation. I half-expected my left hand to suddenly leap into life, and for the whole day after that first dose, I wandered around the house, periodically sitting at the computer and typing a few lines as a test to see if anything had changed. No changes; no effect.

The doctor warned me about possible side effects, and told me to call him if they were too bad. I took the first dose on a Saturday morning, thinking that if there were going to be problems, I'd see them Saturday or Sunday, and would be on top of it by the workday on Monday. Reasonable, logical, and wrong.

I felt fine all day Saturday, but there were no changes my symptoms.

Sunday, I repeated the process—still no changes in my hand and arm. I went to bed feeling just a little out of sorts on Sunday night.

On Monday morning, the alarm rang at the normal time. I rolled out of bed and promptly fell down as the room turned on its side. I had read that dizziness and disorientation were possible side effects, but this wasn't dizziness. This was a carnival Tilt-a-Whirl ride missing a few important bolts. I decided to relax on the bedroom floor for a few minutes and consider my options.

I discovered I could control the disorientation if I kept my head still and moved very slowly. So, looking like the Tin Man on a rainy day, I made my way to the couch to recover from the process of getting out of bed. After a few minutes, the dizziness faded enough that I could eat. I made several telephone calls—one to my office to let them know I would be working from home, and then to the neurologist to ask, "So, what is THIS nonsense all about?"

He called back later that day, and it was a short conversation:

Me: "I'm very dizzy."

Doc: "Yes. That's one of the potential side effects."

Me: "I'm sorry, I wasn't clear. I'm VERY dizzy."

Doc: "Yes, we discussed this. You may experience some unpleasant side effects at first. They will likely fade over time. It's important that we determine how well you respond to medication."

Me: "Dizzy. Very dizzy."

Doc: "Is there anything else? No? Feel free to call anytime."

I had started down the path that all people with Parkinson's, or PWPs, walk: the balancing act between the benefits of various treatments and the unavoidable side effects that can be worse than the disease. And this was just the first few days of a simple drug challenge to validate the diagnosis.

The dizziness eventually eased, but the benefits did not appear. After six weeks, I visited the neurologist again and reported the news. And over the next three months, the pattern repeated with a succession of drugs. Most caused violent nausea and vomiting with every dose. I had side effects by the truckload, but I was still not seeing any noticeable benefits. I had the same stiffness, slowness, unsteadiness, and lack of fine motor control.

After a very unpleasant trial with a new drug, I called the doctor's office again. I needed information. The drugs don't appear to be working; what does this mean? Is the diagnosis a mistake? Do I have a brain tumor after all, or do I just need a better diet? The doctor called back quickly, and as I stood on the outside patio of a local restaurant, he gave me his rundown.

I clearly had the symptoms of Parkinson's disease, but the cause was unknown. It didn't appear that I was responding to medication—that was called drug-unresponsive Parkinsonism. There were several possible culprits. "Space-occupying defects" in my brain had been ruled out, as had several other unusual possibilities. There was something called "atypical Parkinsonism" that could be responsible. Only time would tell. We would have to wait.

Unfamiliar technical-sounding terms are irresistible to me, so I hit the web again. This time I wanted more detail, so I went to the Mayo Clinic website. I found new information about atypical Parkinsonism: the common characteristic is a rapid degeneration of physical and mental function ending in death.

I was stunned again. Only months ago I was happily unaware, enjoying time with Amy and my kids, teaching scuba diving on weekends, learning a new job, and living a normal life. Today, I "would have to wait" to find out if I had a disease that would quickly steal my health, my body, my mind, and, finally, my life. In desperation, I sought another medical opinion.

I searched throughout the country for the best neurologists for a second opinion. There were multiple options, including road trips to the Mayo Clinic(s), Washington, Cleveland, Houston, Dallas, and many other places. There were excellent options in San Antonio, though, and I had learned enough to know I wanted to see a movement disorder specialist, so I made an appointment.

During my first appointment, the doctor listened patiently as I gave him a quick synopsis, and he asked a number of pointed and probing questions about my medications, my symptoms, and my history. He asked questions that I found a little strange, such as, "does your arm or hand ever do things on its own, or feel like it doesn't belong to you?" and then administered another hokey-pokey exam, this one more comprehensive than any other. I walked up and down, tapped, dragged, clenched, touched, and twisted as directed, wishing for a little music to make my timing better. He also snuck up behind me and pulled on my shoulders suddenly—I didn't realize at the time that it was part of the exam, and just thought he had a unique way of interacting with his patients.

We then sat down for a discussion. He was clear, straightforward, and direct.

"Well. It's apparent to me that you have Parkinsonian symptoms, and they're markedly asymmetric, which raises questions. There are some possibilities we have to rule out, so here's what we're going to do…"

I left his office with an order for another test to make sure all the useful parts of my brain were getting enough blood, an order for a test with an interesting specimen collection process (I'll never again trust a bottle of apple juice in the refrigerator), an additional blood test to eliminate several metabolic possibilities, and a particularly detailed day-by-day plan for conducting a drug challenge with the right Parkinson's drug. He was clear that, given my history, I would probably have nausea and vomiting problems from the medication, but that I should just bear it as well as I could.

He was absolutely right on all counts—the brain scan showed no blood flow abnormalities in my brain, and the other tests showed nothing more significant than a Vitamin D deficiency. All that remained was to judge my response to medication.

For some PWPs, response to the medicine is like flipping a switch; the effects are quick and obvious. They were assuredly quick and obvious for me: horrible nausea and vomiting after every dose. The doctor made some changes to my daily regimen that made a radical difference, and I embarked on a long, slow, nausea-free increase in dosage. After two months of pills and uncertainty, I went back to my new neurologist for another hokey-pokey exam.

He concluded that I showed significant improvement in motor function. He guessed that my previous violent reaction didn't leave enough medication in my system to have an impact, and that the right combination of drugs made all the difference.

After almost twenty years of slowly growing symptoms and fifteen years of physical disability, I finally had an answer: young-onset idiopathic drug-responsive Parkinson's disease. Even this was only a provisional diagnosis, the result of a winnowing process that had ruled out other conclusions. I learned from my frantic research that even the most careful PD diagnosis was only about 75% accurate, so I had to ask, "Is it possible that this isn't really even Parkinson's?" His response brought the stark reality of my new situation clearly into focus.

"You need to understand that if you don't have Parkinson's disease, the only other possibilities are much worse."

I had been a normal, healthy middle-aged man with some unexplained soreness and stiffness only weeks before. Now, the best I could hope for was life with an incurable, degenerative neurological disease. I was devastated, and had a completely new set of unanswered questions. How could I fight back? What could I do to control this new reality? What should I do next?

PREPARATION

By the time I was fifteen, I had almost convinced myself that the abuse hadn't really happened. It had stopped several years before, and it was such an unbelievable and horrible anomaly that I coped by ignoring it. I tried once to tell my brother Ken, but he was only a teenager himself and simply didn't know what to do with the information. I let it drop, and didn't bring it up again until many years later.

From the outside, my junior high and high school years appeared normal; I was prone to nightmares and anxieties, but I had friends, played sports, and made good if not outstanding grades. The secret I carried, and my belief that I was not only at fault but also faulty in general, sank below the surface; not to heal and disappear, but to fester and wait for the future.

I was tagged as a gifted and talented student in elementary school, and although I was happy with the perceived achievement, I was uncomfortable with being singled out. As I grew older, I developed a love-hate relationship with my academic ability. I was smart, but I hated for adults to comment on it in front of other kids. It made me feel peculiar, and I needed no additional reason to feel different.

I enjoyed the feeling of power that being the "smart kid" gave me, though. I craved the sense of control that knowing the answers gave me, and it came naturally. I was curious about everything, and one of my favorite pastimes was to choose one volume of our World Book Encyclopedia, starting with "A" and continuing through "X-Y-Z," and read it cover to cover. I must have read the entire encyclopedia a dozen times between the ages of eight and fourteen, one letter at a time. The World Book helped me develop an appreciation for the value and power of knowledge, even if many of the facts I learned from its pages were wrong, as I've discovered over the years.

Although I needed the power that academic achievement gave me, it was at odds with another powerful drive: my need to hide. I felt defective and wrong in a way I couldn't define, and I felt much safer and more secure when no one noticed me. These two forces were in constant opposition inside me—I craved the spotlight and the sense of accomplishment and approval it brought, but I also wanted to stay in the shadows.

As an outgrowth of the love of reading and books I received from my sister Kathy, I became a science fiction fan. I immersed myself in tales of spaceships, space exploration, and the steely-eyed, square-jawed heroes who could both out-think and out-shoot bug-eyed monsters and space pirates. As I lost myself in those created worlds, I developed a future vision of myself that combined my intellect with an air of power, fearlessness, and bravery. I wanted to be Virgil Samms, First Lensman of The Galactic Patrol, but I decided that I could settle for being an astronaut. I resolved to become the person I imagined I could be—smart, but strong; a thinker and a doer; equally comfortable at the blackboard or in the cockpit. I wanted to be Alan Shepard, Neil Armstrong, and a less wimpy Luke Skywalker combined.

I developed The Plan. First, I would obtain an appointment to the Air Force Academy and earn a degree in engineering. I would become an Air Force fighter pilot and test pilot. I would eventually earn a Ph.D. in either engineering or physics, and then be assigned to NASA as an astronaut. I resolved to be the first man on Mars.

I gleefully ignored the fact that I became violently carsick on our occasional drives through the mountains in the Shenandoah National Park, and that I had never met a roller coaster that didn't make me vomit. I was on a mission, and naysayers be damned.

I had played baseball, football and basketball when I was younger, but I chose track as my sport in high school. I was a sprinter and quarter-miler, and I was fast enough to compete well and win regularly. My SAT scores were excellent, my grades were good, I didn't have any juvenile felonies on my record, and I cleaned up reasonably well, so an appointment to the Air Force Academy seemed possible.

I completed the Academy application and received nominations from my senators and congressmen. My Academy liaison officer informed me I was a shoo-in, so I decided to have confidence and didn't apply at any other academies or universities. And so, of course, the appointment went to a football player from my high school who also applied, a nice guy who left the Academy under duress during his sophomore year as a result of a youthful indiscretion that involved a young lady and some unusual behavior at a local dance hall. Or so I heard.

Shocked, discouraged, and without much time, I conducted a quick survey of possibilities. I had been offered a track scholarship to Brown University in Rhode Island, but I still wanted to pursue a degree in aerospace engineering and follow The Plan; Brown, although an excellent choice, wasn't much of an engineering school. I was months past the application deadline for most other top-tier engineering schools, so I looked at state schools in Texas and Maryland, the two states where I could claim residency. After rejecting Texas A&M University (mostly because my father recommended it), I enrolled at The University of Texas at Austin and joined Air Force ROTC. I obtained an AFROTC scholarship after my first semester, and after four years as a Longhorn, I earned a degree in aerospace engineering, a promise of a place in Air Force Undergraduate Pilot Training after graduation, and commission as an Air Force Second Lieutenant. I also met my future wife at UT, which, in retrospect, is the best thing I did during my college years.

My entry onto active duty was delayed several months after graduation. I spent the delay working at General Dynamics in Forth Worth on the F-16 fighter and exercising my new American Express card for dinners with my future wife. Finally, I departed for Undergraduate Pilot Training in Columbus, Mississippi. After a minor ripple in The Plan, I was on my way, I thought.

Boy, was I wrong.

WHERE ARE ALL THE GOOD ALTERNATIVES?

I was confused and frustrated during my long journey to a Parkinson's disease diagnosis, but I was satisfied to finally have an answer. After years of wondering, I now had a label and could develop a plan of attack. I was relieved until reality set in.

Dr. Elisabeth Kubler-Ross described grieving as a five-stage process: denial, anger, bargaining, depression, and acceptance. I've been in all five of those places, sometimes on the same day. It's not a steady progression, and I'm not finished yet. Although Parkinson's disease shortens expected lifespan, it's not a directly fatal disease. Many people with Parkinson's live long lives after diagnosis, with slow progression and years of good function. Unfortunately, although the speed of progression and the details are different for everyone, the direction and result is always the same.

Parkinson's is both complex and very simple—it's all about "on" and "off." For a PWP who's on, the various medications and treatments are working as well as they ever do, the symptoms are at a minimum (although never gone), and life is manageable. During off time, though, the full weight of the disease comes crashing down and nothing works. Our arms and legs don't move or move too much, our hands shake or are immobile, our bodies scream with the pain of rigid muscles that won't relax, we shuffle, freeze, and fall, we struggle to eat, to speak, to sleep, to stay awake… in short, on is good, off is bad. Daily life for a PWP is a constant battle to maximize on time, minimize off time, and predict the transitions from one to the other. It's a full-time job, and it can be exhausting, frightening, and discouraging. Parkinson's steals not only the ability to move and communicate effectively, but it also damages self-esteem, destroys relationships, halts promising careers in mid-stride, and sentences both PWPs and their loved ones to a seemingly eternal cycle of medication, daily struggles with the basic activities of living, and a slow decline in spite of heroic efforts. A friend and fellow PWP once told me that Parkinson's is "like being stuck on the railroad tracks in front of a slow-moving train— you know it's coming, but even though it takes years to arrive, you can't get out of the way and you can't make it stop."

After my diagnosis, I adjusted the medications and fought my way through debilitating side effects just as every other PWP does. I lost friends I had known for years who stopped responding to attempts at communication, and I made many new friends in many places. My family and I also tried to manage the fear, uncertainty, and anxiety that accompany a progressive, incurable illness. How long would I be able to continue functioning? What would happen when I couldn't work anymore? How fast would the disease progress? How would our family change? Would we be okay?

It quickly became clear that I was unusually affected by side effects from PD medications. Nausea, dizziness, disorientation, fatigue, insomnia, sleep attacks, hallucinations, compulsive behavior, dyskinesia—they were all a part of my PD experience. Since PD is not well understood, the drugs used to relieve the symptoms often cause as many problems as they solve.

Sleep disruptions and hallucinations were particular problems for me. I had had occasional bouts of insomnia prior to being diagnosed, but when I began taking a particular PD medication, I learned what insomnia really is. I would regularly be unable to sleep at night for two or three nights in a row, and even when I did sleep, it was not for more than an hour or two at a time. I tried a variety of sleep medications, but although they helped me sleep slightly longer, I would awaken unrefreshed, disoriented, and sluggish.

It wasn't as if I couldn't catch occasional catnaps, though. I had sleep attacks—sudden, uncontrollable sleepiness during the day. I fell asleep in meetings, during meals, and during one-on-one conversations. In the past, I had occasionally fallen asleep during lectures or business presentations, but it was a new experience to fall asleep during a presentation where I was the one speaking. I imagine it was novel experience for the audience also.

I also fell asleep behind the wheel. I had enough warning to pull into a parking lot or to the side of the road before the uncontrollable sleepiness overtook me, but it was dangerous and disconcerting. I fell asleep several times at stoplights, and only woke up when the irritated drivers behind me blew their horns. Once, I woke up from one of these short naps to a concerned woman knocking on my car window. I rolled down the window.

"Are you okay? Do you need an ambulance?"

"No, thanks," I responded. "I'm just a little sleepy."

"Well, maybe you shouldn't be driving, then, hmm? Why don't you get off the road before you kill yourself or someone else?"

I debated telling her about Parkinson's disease, dopamine agonists, and sleep attacks, but decided that this really wouldn't be the right time for an awareness and education session. Besides, I wasn't sure I could make it through the discussion without falling asleep again.

I also hallucinated. I had never had this particular experience before, so the first time that I saw a squirrel run across the living room floor, I was startled and shocked. We had a backyard full of squirrels, and I enjoyed watching them steal seed from the bird feeder in the mornings and fight with the birds. I thought, "Oh, great. I left the door open—how am I going to get that tree-rat out of here?" I spent thirty minutes trying to find the damned thing in the house, with the cat sitting on the couch watching me with patient contempt. Our cat, a huge Siamese that tolerated no nonsense from anyone or anything, was a serial killer of birds and squirrels, and ruled the house from the couch like a furry dictator.

I saw the squirrel again from the corner of my eye, and glanced over at the cat—he gazed back at me as if to say, "Yes? Is there something you can do for me?" I was astounded that this killer didn't see the squirrel and make it pay for its impudence. When I saw several more small furry animals running just out of clear eyesight across the floor and the cat didn't react, I began to suspect that maybe they weren't really there.

Over the next two years, the sleep problems and hallucinations became slowly worse. One memorable evening, I was sitting sleepless at about 3:00 AM, writing an email to a friend, when I had an eerie sense that someone was standing behind me and looking over my shoulder. I looked quickly and was grateful I didn't see anyone, but the feeling didn't go away. From that time on, I have had the pervasive feeling that there is someone standing behind me, just out of view. I habitually check over my shoulder. Although I know that it is a hallucination, it is upsetting and disconcerting.

I also heard whispering just out of earshot; the sound of people talking quietly in the next room. The long nights of insomnia were lonely, but now I felt like I was living through my own personal version of "The Shining," complete with ghosts moving in the shadows, small furry creatures scurrying across the floor, and barely perceptible whispering from the next room. I have never reached the point of delusion where I believe that these manifestations are real, but it is a wholly unwelcome experience anyway.

I had reached the point where my high medication dosage caused unacceptable side effects, and attempting to decrease the dosage resulted in unacceptable symptom control. My neurologist recommended that I consider a surgical treatment: deep brain stimulation (DBS) surgery.

When he suggested the idea for the first time, I had only been diagnosed for about two years. I said, "You've got to be kidding—that's for late-stage Parkinson's, after everything else stops working, isn't it?" I apparently have a limitless capacity for being wrong, and I was this time, too. DBS actually works best for people who are still benefiting from medication, but with unacceptable side effects. It also works best for people who are relatively early in the disease, who don't have other complications or significant cognitive impacts, and who are not falling often. In other words, me.

So, after weighing the risk factors and evaluating the data, I decided to have DBS surgery in June 2011. The surgery required preparation—a full-anesthesia MRI for brain mapping, a neuropsychological test to make sure I wasn't demented enough to be a bad surgical risk, and a "putting my affairs in order" process. We're talking brain surgery here, after all. Even though the likely outcome was positive, there were major risks, and my family and I had to prepare for all possibilities. My typical approach of hoping for the best and preparing for the worst gained a new intensity.

Hope is good—it provides the courage to press forward even in the face of fear and uncertainty. I was afraid of the procedure, but I was encouraged by my neurologist who always tells me the truth even when it stings, and by many fellow PWPs who had braved their own fear and apprehension with good results. Amy and the kids supported me also; they were willing to do whatever it took to give me a chance at a better quality of life even if none of us knew what that meant. With that going for me, a little brain surgery seemed like a good risk.

AVIATION

I'd arrived at Columbus Air Force Base, Mississippi in the fall of 1984, full of determination and ready to be an Air Force pilot. I had been slightly diverted on Step One of The Plan, but I had found an outstanding alternative; who but a Texas Aggie wouldn't want to be a Texas Longhorn? I had also met the love of my life. The future looked bright.

Pilot training commenced with physical training and academics, and I quickly found that my bachelor's degree in aerospace engineering wasn't an asset. Rather than discussing the lift equation that governs an airplane in flight, I learned that airplanes flew because of the "lifties" on the wings. When you turned, the lifties rolled off the wings, and that's why you had to add power and pull on the stick to stay level. So much for Bernoulli, Navier, and Stokes—all pinheads without silver wings. I decided I could live with that—I was certain flight test school would be different.

Finally the long-awaited day arrived—my first flight in an Air Force jet trainer. In 1984, Air Force student pilots flew in the T-37B and the T-38, and my "dollar ride" was in the left seat of a T-37B Dragonfly. That's not what the aircraft was really called, of course. The T-37 was a "Tweet," or, if you were wordy, a "6000-pound bird whistle."

I had passed the Air Force Reserve Officer Training Corps Flight Instruction Program in college, which was designed to give cadets headed for the cockpit enough small-aircraft flight hours before Air Force pilot training to limit the likelihood of sheer incompetence or unresolvable lack of coordination. I did well in FIP in a small plane, but here was the real thing—a twin-engine jet aircraft. My dream was coming true. With my flight suit, parachute, helmet, and oxygen mask, I thought I had died and gone to heaven. Later (1.3 hours later, according to my logbook), I was sure I had died, but I was no longer sure I was in heaven.

The official purpose of the dollar ride, named for the silver dollar each student was expected to pay the instructor for his or her first flight, was to introduce a new pilot-training student to the aerospace environment. Unofficially, the instructors competed to see if they could make their students airsick. Never one to disappoint, I puked enthusiastically. We all laughed, and the dozen or so of us who left the flight line that day carrying white plastic bags caught a little good-natured teasing, but no one held it against us.

We usually flew three training missions a day, interspersed with simulator time and academics, and the days were long. Report time in the flight room was 2:30 AM during early week, and 4:30 AM during late week. A duty day was twelve hours long—a perfect environment for someone living out their calling and preparing for what they were born to do. Unfortunately, I learned over the next six months that, in addition to whatever else I was destined to do, I had been born to heave.

My problem was complicated by the weather in Columbus and my predisposition to ear and sinus infections. Whenever I gained ground on the airsickness, I would come down with an ear infection and be placed by the flight surgeon on non-flying status. I would typically be grounded for a week or so, which was just long enough to lose my progress in controlling the airsickness. I developed a pattern and a reputation, but I was determined to fight through it.

Airsickness in pilot training fell into two broad categories—it was either an unavoidable physical characteristic of a particular student's inner ear and brain, or it was something they euphemistically called "manifestation of apprehension," or MOA. The distinction was important—they were willing to work with physical problems, but with MOA, the Air Force was uninterested in even allowing the student to remain on active duty. They determined the difference with dexscope.

Dexscope is a combination of the drugs Dexedrine and scopolamine. Scopolamine numbs the inner ear and makes motion sickness effectively impossible, at the cost of severe drowsiness. It's also called the "zombie drug," and in larger doses can cause agitation, delusions, psychosis, and hallucinations. Dexedrine is, well… speed. It keeps you very awake and crispy, makes your skin crawl and your eyeballs itch, and gives you an overwhelming desire to talk fast on the radio. Truly a combination made for the high-speed aerospace environment.

Someone taking dexscope could be strapped in a roller coaster upside down eating raw buzzard all afternoon and feel fine, but if fear and anxiety caused the sickness, dexscope didn't help at all. The flight surgeon decided to try dexscope.

I flew three missions on dexscope, and they were the most sublimely wonderful aviation experiences of my life. I felt free and limitless; the aircraft went where I told it to, and I felt like I was wearing it rather than sitting inside it. Loops, spins, cloverleafs, barrel rolls, Immelmanns, chandelles, split-s's—for so long I had wanted them to be beautiful and effortless, and now they were. The sky was blue, the clouds were puffy, and

I could even understand the radio. I was finally in heaven. I was heavily medicated and I was sure I could feel my hair growing, but I wasn't airsick.

The experiment satisfied the flight surgeon and squadron commander. I wasn't one of those MOA types, so they were willing to give me the benefit of the doubt. They were clear, though—one more episode of post-solo airsickness, and I was done. I think I might have been fine if not for yet another ear infection.

When I recovered a week later, I flew one dual mission with my instructor to make sure I hadn't forgotten everything, and then I went up solo on a mission to practice aerobatics. Unfortunately, I actually tried to practice aerobatics, and that was my downfall.

I took off uneventfully and proceeded to my assigned practice area, a pie-shaped wedge of sky defined by distance and heading from the navigation beacon at the base. I arrived without incident and flew a couple of experimental Immelmanns and loops—a few twinges of nausea, but not too bad. I decided to push a little and I set up for a cloverleaf—four loops with a ninety-degree turn near the top of each loop. I remembered how much fun it was when I was heavily drugged, and I wanted to see if could do it without benefit of pharmaceuticals.

I was at the top of the third leaf when I felt a familiar sensation—it was time to hurl. I was disappointed, but I had been through this before and I was a pro, I thought. I was drifting lazily over the top of the loop as I twisted slightly in the ejection seat to reach the supply of white plastic bags in my flight suit leg pocket. I was below stall speed, but I was almost weightless and the airplane didn't notice, even though my inner ear protested violently.

As I twisted to reach the bag and slapped the mask off my face to do what came unnaturally, my leg slipped and I kicked the right rudder. Hard. Below stall speed, upside down, nearly weightless. I should have had better sense (aerospace engineer and all that), but I was young and stupid. The aircraft lurched, and in reflex and inexperience I jerked back on the stick and stalled. The aircraft stopped flying and started falling. Before I could even think, "oh, s**t, that was dumb," I was involved in my first, last, and only inadvertent inverted spin.

Emergency procedures are a critical part of Air Force pilot training, and some emergency procedures are important enough that they print them in large block letters in your checklist and make you memorize them. They're called "boldface procedures" and spin recovery was a boldface procedure. I still remember it:
1. THROTTLES – IDLE
2. RUDDER AND AILERONS – NEUTRAL
3. STICK – ABRUPTLY FULL AFT AND HOLD
4. RUDDER – ABRUPTLY APPLY FULL RUDDER OPPOSITE

SPIN DIRECTION (OPPOSITE TURN NEEDLE) AND HOLD

5. STICK – ABRUPTLY FULL FORWARD ONE TURN AFTER APPLYING RUDDER

6. CONTROLS – NEUTRAL AND RECOVER FROM DIVE

I had completely forgotten about my need to vomit, and was instead focused on my need not to plummet to the ground and end my life in fiery embarrassment. I had forgotten everything else, and couldn't have even told you my own name, but I remembered that boldface. It must have worked, because I found myself in level flight again, muttering the same obscenity over and over. I now had time to puke; this time, it might have been a manifestation of apprehension.

All this excitement occurred in the first twenty minutes of a planned, 1.3-hour mission, but my zeal for aerobatics had cooled. I extended the speed brake and flew back and forth in the training area, burning fuel and thinking about my future. My thoughts ranged between extremes, from, " I can play this off—maybe no one saw me," to, " I should probably just eject now, walk back to Texas, and get a job at a gas station." When I had burned enough fuel to give me options, I headed back to the base for the last landing of my military aviation career.

The supervisor of flying and the squadron commander were waiting for me. They summoned me as soon as I had put my helmet and parachute away. The SOF spoke first.

"Lieutenant King, how was your mission?" he said.

"Not bad, sir," I said. No blood, I thought.

"Question for you, Lieutenant. Is a spin an authorized solo maneuver?"

"No, sir, it's not."

"Then what the hell did you think you were doing out there solo, spinning my jet?"

Before I answered, I thought about my dream of being an astronaut, my reluctance to show weakness, my desire not to quit or look foolish, and my practical need to have a job so I could marry the girl I had fallen in love with (and, much less importantly, to pay for the new sports car I had bought). I compared those things to being dead, and answered, "Sir, it was an accident. I was airsick, and…" The unvarnished truth came out. I was never a good liar, and they knew what had happened anyway. The crew chief had seen my little white bag.

The squadron commander finally spoke. He said, "Son, go see the flight surgeon," and with those words, my Air Force flight career and my aspirations for glory in space were over. They were over long before that, actually; I just refused to see the truth.

IT LOOKS LIKE AN INK BLOT

My decision in the spring of 2011 to have DBS surgery was difficult, but there's nothing easy about any of the elements of this disease. There are always tough decisions, trade-offs, and hard choices between unpleasant options.

Two facts complicated the decision: the fact that I was very young (forty-eight is young, isn't it?), and the fact that I had only been diagnosed for two years. Those two facts recurred in conversations about my decision to have the surgery. "REALLY? You're having brain surgery? On purpose? You look fine to me—why would you want to do that?"

Most PWPs must repeatedly address the last comment, even with family members and close friends. On some days we do look and feel better than on others, and we're grateful for those days. It was difficult for me to know how to respond to those well-meaning comments. It didn't seem right to say, "Thanks very much for saying that; however, let's not forget that I'm not better, I'm not going to get better, and tomorrow I'm going to look terrible again." There's a fine line between reminding people that PD is variable, capricious, and incurable, and just accepting a nice compliment and the good wishes and concerns that lie behind it at face value. It reminded me of the Saturday Night Live skits that feature Debbie Downer—she never had anything good to say. It tends to stifle conversation when you feel the need to say, "Yes, it is an absolutely beautiful day, and I've never seen the sky so blue and the sun so bright. I have Parkinson's disease, you know."

Those two facts, coupled with the fact that I sometimes appeared to be unaffected by the disease, troubled me as I weighed the pros and cons, sifted through the mountains of available information, and talked to dozens of patients, doctors, experts, family members, and friends. I was young for DBS surgery. Although DBS is now being used more often for younger patients, one of my neurosurgeon's nursing staff mentioned that I was the youngest person she had seen to have the surgery. In addition, I had only been diagnosed for a short time; many people who have this disease manage their symptoms and treatments well for years, and have no interest in or need for DBS.

Sleep disturbances were the main problems that drove me toward DBS. I hoped that DBS would eventually help me taper the amount of medication I was taking, reduce side effects, and help me sleep, and not just in the car driving to work in the morning.

The first step was easy: a two-hour full-anesthesia MRI. I only remember the smiling faces in the MRI room, the IV in my arm, and a chemically-induced black curtain that came down momentarily and then came up again in the recovery room. The nurse said, "Well, welcome back. How are you feeling?"

Blearily, I responded, "I think I was abducted by aliens for a moment."

I experienced no ill effects and no post-anesthesia complications. The detailed map of my brain the neurosurgeon obtained allowed him to plan a precise implantation path for the DBS electrodes, avoid some of my favorite parts of my brain, and finish in exactly the right spot in my subthalamic nucleus. I didn't even know I had a subthalamic nucleus until then.

According to my neurosurgeon, DBS is not a difficult procedure to perform. The key to success is to perform the procedure exactly the same way every time, with the same equipment and the same processes, in the same order, with the same team, carefully and without fanfare. He told me he wasn't interested in being famous, writing journal articles on new processes, or trying all the latest equipment. He just wanted to perform every procedure with predictably excellent results. Coupled with his experience level (well over 1000 successful implantations at this point), his approach made my choice of surgeons easy.

The next step was a neuropsychological exam. Some people are better candidates for DBS surgery than others, and one of the major contraindications for DBS is dementia. The neuropsych exam looks for signs of dementia, and also sets a baseline for cognitive function, memory, coordination, and spatial orientation. With this information, we could compare my pre-surgery state with post-surgery, and see both improvement and decline.

The surgery was scheduled for June 9, 2011, and would last for three to four hours. I would actually be awake for about half of the procedure. I had heard that the brain itself has no pain receptors; I thought that was a fascinating concept. I was more concerned about the process of getting to the brain, though. Past experience with wildly pitched baseballs, tree branches, cave ceilings, and open kitchen cabinets made me quite confident that my scalp and skull enjoyed no such freedom from pain. I hoped the surgeon had thought of that.

I had researched the procedure and talked to other patients, so I thought

I knew what to expect. I would arrive at the hospital early on the ninth and receive a new look—I would have my head shaved, a new experience for me. I couldn't recall having seen my own scalp before, except for brief periods in the Air Force when I was overenthusiastic at the barbershop. After the shaving, the surgical team would then install a stereotactic frame—a metal ring that would be screwed into the bone of my skull to keep my head completely still during the procedure. A brain scan to validate my alien-abduction MRI would follow, as a double check that I hadn't done something to change my brain and to verify that the surgical plan was still correct.

I would then proceed to the operating room, where I hoped they kept the serious painkillers. The surgical team would open up my scalp, drill into my skull, and implant two electrical leads in my brain, following the predetermined path. I would be awake, perhaps so I could provide color commentary and tell jokes. After they determined that all was well and everything was where it should be, they would finally let me sleep. I was looking forward to that part of the procedure.

They would anchor the electrodes to plastic plugs in my skull connected to long electrical leads. Those leads would be placed under the skin of my scalp, neck, and upper chest, and terminate in a new battery pack and stimulation computer implanted under the skin of my upper chest below my collarbone. After I healed, the only visible signs would be a slight bulge in my upper chest and two small bulges on the top of my head. I would spend two weeks recovering from the procedure, and then after six to eight weeks, my neurologist would program the device. After tuning and adjustment, I would be a new, electrified man.

My work colleagues thought my surgery might be a unique opportunity to push the boundaries of science and experiment with the man-machine interface. In the lab I helped to manage, we developed ways to make complex technical systems do things their designers didn't intend (we didn't use the term "hacker"—it's rude and inaccurate). We took our work seriously, and I had the sense some of my team took it too seriously. I learned to smile and nod at the comments about the "Six Million Dollar Man," questions like "so, will you be Borg after this? Will we be assimilated?" and even my new nickname, "One of One," a play on "Seven of Nine," a half-robot/half-human character from one of the Star Trek TV shows. However, I drew the line at questions like, "What did you say the control system signal looked like? Do you know anything about the effective range of control? What kind of processor is in the stimulation system? Do you mind dropping by the lab for a few minutes when the system is installed? We'd like to test a theory." Engineers are just hilarious, in an incomprehensible kind of way.

In May 2011, I completed a major milestone on the way to the surgery date. I didn't know what to expect from the neuropsychological exam, but like many parts of the process, it was fascinating. The exam lasted about three hours, and started with a Minnesota Multiphasic Personality Inventory (MMPI), a delightful collection of 576 questions that, if you were not already disturbed, could easily make you that way. I had an easy time with questions like, "I often hear voices that tell me to do things I shouldn't do," and, "Demons often inhabit my body." I knew the right answers, regardless of what the truth might actually be. I had a little more trouble with questions like, "I believe I would like the work of a forest ranger," and, "I believe I would enjoy being a woman." I may have overthought some of the questions; surely, it depends on which forest ranger and which woman, doesn't it?

There were many other tests in the neuropsych exam. Most of them activated my sense of competitiveness, and I worked hard. It was clear to me, however, that on some segments I didn't do well, and I wondered whether it was just a normal effect of growing older or whether it was Parkinson's disease. One of the tests involved saying as many words that started with a particular letter as I could in one minute. Piece of cake, I thought. I completed F and N without any problems, and then came the letter A. I started off strong; "apple, aardvark, archive, argument," and then stalled. I couldn't think of a single word that started with "A." I had an intense dialogue with myself trying to break through the A-word logjam, but that entire section of the dictionary had disappeared.

"Oh, come on, there're all kinds of words that start with A. How about... no, I used that one. Now, there's... no, not that one—too vulgar. Well, there's... no, that's a proper noun, and he said I couldn't use those. I wonder if he'd notice if I just got up and left the room? How long IS one minute, anyway? This is just getting ridiculous now. A, A, come on—you're a smart guy—please, just one more..."

"Time's up," the psychologist said.

"Oh, thank God," I said. "What just happened?"

In typical psychologist form, he said, "What do YOU think just happened?" I fought an internal battle with myself, and avoided ruining the whole test by strangling him. It's the small victories that are the most satisfying.

One of the final tests involved dozens of cards printed with different numbers of colored shapes. My task was to match the cards and figure out what the rules were for matching. My inquisitor laid four cards face-up on the table and gave me the rest of the deck.

"You place the cards where you think they go, one at a time, and after each one I'll tell you whether it's correct or incorrect." Great, I thought. I'm good at this kind of thing.

I started slapping cards down confidently. It went well, briefly.

"Let's see—three green squares. Does that go with the two green triangles, the one blue square, or the three red circles? Let's try… the circles," I thought.

"Correct."

"Ah. Numbers. Now, one yellow triangle ought to go with one red square…"

"Correct," he said again.

"Way too easy," I thought. Confidently, I continued to slap the cards down, receiving each "correct" as my due reward for being so darned smart. I placed three yellow circles on three red triangles, and was already reaching for the next card when I heard him say, "That's incorrect."

"Huh? No, it's not."

"I'm sorry, but it is incorrect," he said. "Okay," I thought. "I just have to revise the algorithm a little bit. New data; no big deal. Numbers go with numbers, unless there's a match of colors and shapes. So, three yellow circles go with any number of yellow circles first, then any card with three of anything. Got it…"

"Correct, correct, correct, incorrect." WHAT???

"Okay, another revision… shapes plus colors, then numbers, then colors alone, but only if… no, wait. Shapes, then colors, but only if there isn't a shape-color match, or if there are more than six cards in my hand, or if it's Tuesday and not a leap year… no, wait." My mind was awash with nested if-then loops, conditional rules, cases, and other logical constructs that my software development colleagues lived and breathed, but that I only vaguely remembered from my one software engineering class in graduate school. My tendency to over-think didn't occur to me then. There was a mystery here, and I was going to figure it out.

"Correct, correct, correct, incorrect, incorrect, incorrect, incorrect, incorrect, incorrect, incorrect, incorrect, incorrect, correct…"

"Can we go back to the "A" words now, please?"

Whenever I thought I finally understood the rule set, he said, "that's incorrect." I suspected that this wasn't about placing cards, but instead about judging my tolerance for frustration. I resolved to be imperturbable.

"Correct, incorrect, incorrect, incorrect, incorrect, incorrect, incorrect, incorrect, incorrect, incorrect…"

"Oh, come on. Now you're just messing with me."

In his best Sigmund Freud voice, he said, "Hmmmm. Do you often think that people are messing with you? What do they do to mess with you? Does everyone mess with you?" Again the internal struggle, again a small victory. He lived, and I stayed out of jail.

After roughly ten years in hell, I finally came to the end of the card deck. I pushed back slightly from the table, looked my new friend in the eye, and said, "Okay. What's the story? How does this work?"

"Well, I'm really not supposed to tell you…"

I debated telling him about my internal struggle, and how we might both lose if he didn't cough up the answer, but I decided that might work against me. In my calmest, most non-psychotic, non-frustrated voice I said, "I think it would be really good for us both if you told me what I wanted to know."

"It's actually pretty simple," he said. "For the first few minutes, you're supposed to match the numbers. Then you're supposed to match the colors, and then you're supposed to match the shapes. You seemed to be having a hard time with that."

I stopped breathing momentarily, and even stopped shaking, which is a significant event for someone with Parkinson's disease.

"You were CHANGING THE RULES? Let's discuss for a moment what a rule actually is, shall we? Let's talk about horses in midstream; let's talk about consistency; let's talk about what you don't do in the middle of a test. Okay? Okay?"

"So, consistency is important to you? Do you expect the world to be consistent? How does it make you feel when people are not consistent? Was your mother consistent?"

Apparently, I passed the test. They didn't cancel my appointment for surgery.

COERCION

The Air Force and I agreed that I could keep my commission if I never again tried to pilot a military jet aircraft. I spent several months in the spring of 1985 working in the Columbus base commander's office as an errand boy while the Powers That Be decided my future. While there, I met a major who had been a flight commander in the student squadron, responsible for a dozen or so instructor pilots and perhaps forty students. He had fallen from grace with the Air Force for some reason, and had been stripped of both his command and his wings. He and I were in a kind of limbo, waiting to learn what our futures held.

I saw him regularly in the cafeteria, so out of politeness I struck up a conversation with him one afternoon.

"Hi, Major. How are things going?"

"Hello, Lieutenant. Have you accepted Christ as your personal Lord and Savior?"

I was taken aback. I stammered, "Well, I'm not sure. I used to got to church, but I haven't had time recently, I was a student here but I washed out for air sickness, my dog ate my homework, I think I hear my mother calling me, I've got to go find anything else to do, sir, goodbye and enjoy your lunch," as I backed toward the door. I probably could have handled the situation more tactfully, but I had never been asked that directly before, and I didn't know what to say. I knew my answer was, "No, and I don't want to hear about it from you, either," but I also sensed that would be the wrong thing to say. I hid in the base historian's office for the rest of the day and hoped I wouldn't see the major again before I left for my new assignment.

Of course, I saw him every day for the next two weeks. I finally tired of ducking into doorways and diving into the shrubbery every time he appeared, so when he approached me in the base library, where I was using my engineering degree to update a section of the base history document, I resigned myself to a conversation I really didn't want to have.

"Hello again, Lieutenant. Do you know Jesus?"

I admitted that I didn't, but that I had gone to church when I was younger. I just didn't see the point any longer.

He began a long, rambling monologue filled with Bible verses, commentary about the nature of sin, personal anecdotes about his conversations with God, and the evil nature of the modern Air Force. He then said, "Are you willing to get down on your knees with me right here and accept Jesus?"

I felt trapped and embarrassed, but I was surprised that I also felt a touch of fear. I remembered that this was how I felt when my father abused me. Trapped, ashamed, frightened of what this crazy person here with me might do, shocked by my belated recognition that he wasn't what I thought he was, wanting to be anywhere else but frozen in place by my perception of his authority over me. An unexpected anger pounded in my temples.

"No, Major, I am not. I'm not interested in your God or anything you have to say. Do you really think you're doing the right thing? You don't know me, sir, and you don't have any right to pressure me like this. If you talk to me again, I'll tell the wing commander and base commander. Leave me alone." I wished I could have kept the quaver out of my voice, but I was both enraged and apprehensive. I didn't know why then, but I also felt a slight sense of liberation that I attributed to telling a senior officer to bug off.

"Lieutenant, my duty is to God, and my mission is to save souls. That's why they want me to leave. You won't be telling them anything they don't already know."

I was dumbfounded, but I was on a roll. "Major, you're making me really uncomfortable. Even if I were interested, and I'm not, bullying me on duty is wrong." In memory, I imagine myself looking like Dirty Harry Callahan, but Barney Fife is probably closer to the truth.

He shook his head. "I'm just trying to save your soul from Hell. That's where you're headed." He walked away.

The only other time I saw him was my last duty day at Columbus, as I was out-processing. I had gone to the base gym to get a signature verifying that I didn't have any of their basketballs in my possession, and I saw him sitting at a desk in the hallway between the men and women's locker rooms. It was his desk, complete with a pencil holder, a telephone, and his nameplate, and he was filling out forms. The leadership at the base was shaming him, because no one wanted him in their organization while they drummed him out of the military. I never learned whether his infraction had only been his inability to reconcile his religious zeal with the responsibility he had accepted with his commission, or whether there was more to it. My indignation had cooled somewhat, but I still thought he deserved everything he was getting; he had turned his back on duty, honor, and country, and used his rank and position to achieve personal goals that didn't have anything to do with his obligation as an officer. I pitied him, but he still disgusted me, and I was sure that he must be seriously mentally deranged.

In retrospect, I overreacted. I was in the grip of forces and motivations I didn't understand but that had bubbled close to the surface for many years. I associated religion with coercion, and coercion with abuse, shame, and guilt. I wanted no part of it, and I began to consciously reject God and religion in any form.

DENYING THE BRUTAL TRUTH

The neuropsychological exam forced me to confront a scary subject I had been avoiding—the cognitive side of Parkinson's disease. I had been focused on the physical symptoms of Parkinson's: the movement symptoms, the autonomic nervous system problems, the degeneration of my body and physical competence. I had been ignoring the other part of this insidious disease: the potential decline of executive function, memory, complex decision-making, multitasking, and other higher-level cognitive abilities. This characteristic of PD was the most disturbing and frightening to me. I relied on my ability to think and to solve problems as part of my profession and of my basic personality; the possibility of losing my mental competence and not "being me" was deeply troubling. The neuropsych exam emphasized that possibility for me. How would I know what was happening if my instrument of observation was compromised? Would I feel it slipping away, like HAL 9000, the computer in the movie *2001: A Space Odyssey?* "My mind is going. I can feel it, Dave. I can feel it. I'm... afraid."

A Parkinson's diagnosis is devastating for the PWP, but in some ways it's actually easier on a PWP than it is on his or her family. Every day, I'm free to choose how I respond to PD, but Amy, my children, and my extended family don't have the same type of freedom. None of us asked for PD, but I have more control than the people who surround me. I dance to the tune PD calls, but I am free to choose how I dance. They not only have to dance with me, they also have to be patient as I lead the dance, and try not to complain when I step on their feet.

My diagnosis was difficult for my whole family, and we all responded differently. After the initial shock, I tried to become a Parkinson's expert. I wanted to know everything about the disease: symptoms, causes, treatments, prognosis, ongoing research, and alternative therapies. I read constantly, and haunted online support groups and chat rooms. It was my normal approach to a threat—using knowledge and information as a weapon. It usually wasn't effective, but it gave me something to do and let me maintain my illusion of control.

I eventually had to step away from my intense focus on learning everything about Parkinson's. It was obsessive, and I focused too much on the horror stories. I threw myself into advocacy instead. I joined a local support group that became a surrogate family for me. I found people who knew what I was going through because they were also going through it. With the support group, I discovered a sense of community and belonging that I craved, and an opportunity for leadership that was particularly satisfying. Leaning on my leadership and management experience from almost thirty years in business and the military, I became the president and board chairman of the local chapter of a national Parkinson's organization. I spoke at support groups, was interviewed on the radio, and even was the subject of a feature story in the local newspaper. Instead of being someone who happened to have the disease, I started to become the disease—it became my identity. I even began wearing a silver representation of a dopamine molecule on a chain around my neck. I can only imagine how irritating I must have been.

Amy, on the other hand, was facing the possibility for the first time in our lives together of having to be the primary breadwinner, and it panicked her. She threw herself into her career and tried to establish a twenty-year foundation over the course of twelve months. She was upset and frightened by the gradual changes she saw in me, and unconsciously began to draw away. We were unable to talk about the details of my disease, make plans for the future, or bond together as a team to meet the challenge. I missed her companionship, but I was in a tailspin myself. I felt guilty and ashamed that my illness and I were the cause of so much upheaval and turmoil in our lives, and knowing how frightened she was, I didn't push.

I needed someone to talk to, and I began to rely on a female friend more than a married man should. I didn't have any conscious evil intent, but I placed myself in a position that could potentially have gotten out of hand, and I didn't even realize I had done it.

Amy and I have been married for almost thirty years now, and we have stood together against challenges large and small. She was there for our children when I was in the Air Force, traveling constantly and never at home even when I was in town. We had lived through periods when we weren't sure where our next meal was coming from, and periods where the activities and priorities of an affluent lifestyle threatened to overcome our better natures. Through it all, we always stood together. Briefly, Parkinson's disease stole that from us.

"For better or worse, in sickness and health, forsaking all others…" These are important words, but they're vastly more than words—they're the core of the strength that has held us together for over a quarter century. They don't just apply to romantic entanglements that can threaten a marriage, but to any relationship that takes on too much importance, regardless of the cause. Parkinson's and all the stresses and baggage it brings tried to steal our strength. Thankfully, Amy and I both recognized it and we fought back. We both received a loud, ringing wake-up call, and just in time. Although there was damage to repair, there was no large-scale destruction, and today we once again stand shoulder-to-shoulder to face the real enemy. The disease will eventually win the war, but it's going to lose this battle.

Not everyone is as blessed as I am. PD is like a wolf tirelessly circling the house, looking for a way in. It not only destroys health, vitality, and life, it also tears families apart, destroys relationships, and can steal the joy from life. The divorce rate for the general population in the US is around fifty percent for first marriages, and somewhat higher for subsequent marriages. For marriages where one spouse is newly diagnosed with PD, however, the divorce rate by some estimates is higher than eighty-five percent. Parkinson's, like other degenerative, chronic diseases, places stress on every element of a relationship, and finds weaknesses that might have gone unnoticed under more normal circumstances. It's a daily battle, and both the enemy and the battlefield change constantly, but we cannot just give up and let it win. Where do you find the strength, however, when just getting out of bed takes all the energy you have?

SERVICE

In late May of 1985, I finally received a new duty assignment and orders for a permanent change of station. I was rebranded as a space operations officer and shipped off to Denver, Colorado for training.

Several months before the nearly spectacular end to my flying career, my girlfriend had become my fiancée, and we settled on June 8, 1985 as the date we would be married. As further evidence that God protects drunks, fools, and unsuccessful pilot candidates, I was ordered to report to Lowry Air Force Base in Denver on June 9, 1985, no later than 1:00 PM. We had time to be married and have a slice of cake with our guests, but just barely. We left Bergstrom Air Force Base in Austin, Texas, where we had decided to hold the wedding, at 5:00 PM on the eighth. We headed to Denver in my sports car, packed to the brim with the accessories of our new life together.

The trip was largely uneventful, except for an incident that I didn't actually see. Being manly, protective, and mindful that our wedding guests were watching, I was driving when we left Austin. At about 1:00 AM on the back roads of west Texas, I could no longer keep my eyes open and Amy volunteered to drive. We swapped places in the car, and I was asleep within seconds.

Some time later (it might have been minutes or weeks; I was like a corpse in the passenger seat), I awoke to a sudden lurch, a loud thump, and Amy's screams. I was covered in black wetness from the coffee she was drinking while she drove.

"What happened? Are we dead?" I slurred, trying to focus my eyes through a film of sleep and coffee.

"We hit something," she said.

"No… kidding," I responded, remembering at the last moment that we had only been married a matter of hours, and perhaps my new wife wouldn't appreciate my sarcastic, dry wit right at that moment. "Are you okay? Is the car okay? What do you think it was?" At least I got the order of the questions correct.

"I think it might have been an armadillo," she said.

"Felt more like a water buffalo," I cracked, unable to contain myself. I was right—she didn't appreciate my wit.

We stopped at the next town, Dalhart, Texas, and rented a room in a small motel until the sun rose. The owner was not pleased at all to be dragged from his bed at 3:00 AM by two bedraggled newlyweds, wild-eyed and smelling of coffee and fear-sweat, and I think the room he gave us was actually a storage shed. We didn't notice—we collapsed and slept in our clothes for three hours, then continued on our journey with the rising sun.

We arrived in Denver the next day without further incident, and our lives together and my Air Force career (v2.0) began in earnest. After several months in Denver, we again crossed the country to my first duty assignment in Air Force space operations. I had been assigned to be a crew commander at the East Coast PAVE PAWS ballistic missile warning radar site on Cape Cod. I learned that PAWS stands for "Phased Array Warning System." I have no idea what PAVE stands for ("Pretty Awesome and Very Expensive," perhaps).

My job was to wait patiently for World War III, to calmly report that everything was working correctly (if indeed it was) in the event that my radar actually detected the beginning of World War III, and then to be destroyed along with most everyone else in a radioactive hailstorm of submarine-launched ballistic missiles. You'd think that there wasn't much training required for a job like this, especially parts one and three. Part one came easily for me. I'm naturally patient, and I had a wide streak of fatalism that fit with my role as a professional apocalypse-watcher. Part three came easily enough also—it doesn't take great skill to be vaporized, and I had extensive training in vaporization avoidance. If the bombs began falling, I had a secret plan: I would climb under my desk as I was taught in first grade, and wait the Russians out from there.

Part two actually did require extensive training, however. Even if it is a natural reaction, "Oh God, oh God, we're all going to die," was not an acceptable crew commander response to detection of rising sea-launched ballistic missiles. It was just as likely that detection of a massive Soviet missile attack was an exercise or a system malfunction, and shrieking like a child about it only invited ridicule at the officers' club.

So, we trained. Not only did my crew and I participate in the simulated destruction of the world many hundreds of times, we also handled hundreds of fake fires, floods, hurricanes, tornadoes, power failures, system malfunctions, terrorist attacks, heart attacks, printer paper outages, and swarms of locusts. Pharaoh should have trained with the 6th Missile Warning Squadron; then he wouldn't have been so upset by all those plagues, and he would have kept a flawless, detailed, time-stamped log while they were happening.

Occasionally, the real world intruded on our parade of training catastrophes. I was the crew commander on duty on January 28, 1986, a day when we expected the radar to detect a ballistic missile launch for a scheduled event from Cape Canaveral, Florida. It was my sad duty to repeatedly report "no detection" for the launch of the Space Shuttle Challenger, which exploded seventy-three seconds after liftoff, killing all onboard. Challenger never rose high enough to be detected by our radar.

Military operational environments are often dangerous, with hazards both known and unknown. In the Air Force, the danger inherent in flight and strategic weapon system operations and other combat-related activities is expected. Pilots, missile crews, forward air controllers, Air Force Special Operations teams, and other front line operators accept the danger every day and still do their jobs, usually without fanfare or thanks. Every other member of the military does as well, but some jobs are more dangerous than others, and the danger and duty to execute in spite of it are not always obvious. That may be why I was surprised the night my missile-warning console tried to kill me.

During the third of four midnight-to-8:00AM shifts in my crew's duty rotation, about three months before the end of my duty tour on Cape Cod, my crew was working quietly, following one of our innumerable training exercises. The two junior crewmembers were busy tracking high-interest satellites, and my crew chief and I were chatting about our performance on the exercise and listening to jazz music. He had an encyclopedic knowledge of jazz, and was telling me a story about how he had met a musician with the improbable name of Mongo Santamaria in New Orleans as a teenager. I was arguing that no such person existed, and if he did, his mother should be ashamed, when I heard a loud BANG, and the operations center began to fill with acrid white smoke.

The PAVE PAWS radar, although one of the most modern in the Air Force at the time, was composed mostly of 1960s-era technology, and the radar display consoles were huge, 500-pound monstrosities with circular green cathode-ray tube screens, packed with analog electronic components. Chief among these components were cylinder-shaped devices called capacitors. They ranged from thimble-sized to the size of oilcans, and were filled with oil that was rich in polychlorinated biphenyl, a toxic chemical. One of the oil can-sized capacitors in my console had exploded and caught fire, and had sprayed my left arm, torso, and legs with hot PCB-laden capacitor oil.

Under other circumstances, the crew and I would have beaten a hasty exit from the ops center. The air was laced with smoke and I was greasy and stank like a Radio Shack set ablaze. But the fire didn't appear to be getting worse, so we used the fire extinguisher on the console and then did what any operations crew does under similar conditions—we ran the checklist.

In military ops, there's a checklist for everything, so we flipped to the right one and began checking off steps. The crew chief and I conferred briefly, and I decided that satellites could go untracked for a while and sent the junior crewmembers out of the ops center. The fire was out, no one was immediately in danger, the fire response team was on the way, and everyone who needed to be notified had been. We had a dilemma, though—it was four in the morning on a Sunday, and we were the only two people on the entire site qualified to respond to a missile warning alert. We fully expected the Powers That Be to declare our radar non-operational and let us leave the ops center, but they hadn't done it yet. We sat and waited. We were Cold Warriors, and the Russians were sitting in their giant subs just offshore, waiting for us to leave so they could destroy our country, the American way of life, and freedom in general. We weren't going to let that happen. I may have had an overblown perception of our role in the process.

We had both donned Scott Paks (personal breathing devices) and we looked and sounded like Darth Vader. We sat and waited for the phone to ring. After about two minutes, my crew chief sighed and said, "You know, I really wanted to be a jazz musician..."

It finally occurred to me that I didn't necessarily have to wait for a call, so picked up the phone. I was surprised to note that only six minutes had passed since the loud BANG.

"Missile Warning Center."

"This is Otis. We are OPSCAP RED for a fire in the operations center as of 1022 Zulu." I waited, expecting them to anticipate the punch line.

"Yes? You reported that status at 1024 Zulu." Tough crowd; they didn't take the bait.

"My crew chief and I are sitting in the SOC wearing Scott Paks and watching the gauges drop to zero. Request Missile Warning Center permission to abandon the SOC until the fire teams arrive and declare the site safe."

"Stand by, Otis." Stand by? After thirty seconds that seemed like three hours, he returned.

"Permission granted, Otis. Report status and estimated time to return to operation when able." Cold, man, cold. No Christmas card for YOU next year.

By that time, the squadron commander and operations officer had arrived, the fire team was working, and the physician's assistant was checking my crew and me for burns, smoke inhalation, and signs of toxic chemical exposure. We all had headaches, and I felt sick to my stomach. After the commander and operations officer asked questions about the event and our response, they sent us home.

I was off duty for about a week. During that week, I developed a minor skin rash and had occasional periods of nausea and vomiting. For some reason, the PA was concerned about my liver (perhaps he had heard about some of my off-duty recreational activities), so I had a series of liver function tests as well. I don't recall hearing anything about the tests, so I suppose they were normal. I recovered and went back to work, seemingly unaffected by the incident.

A short time later, I was reassigned from Cape Cod to Shemya Air Force Base, Alaska to command a crew at the COBRA DANE radar station. I had volunteered for the assignment almost nine months before, with the understanding that the Air Force would give me a follow-on assignment to Johnson Space Center in Houston on the military side of the Space Shuttle program. The Challenger disaster effectively ended that program, so there was no follow-on assignment to Houston. Just to demonstrate that they could keep at least half the bargain, the Air Force sent me to Alaska anyway on an unaccompanied remote tour for a year. I left behind any concerns about my toxic exposure as well as a very pregnant, very morning-sick wife who went home to live with her parents while I was away.

My year at Shemya ("It's Not The End Of The World, But You Can See It From Here," say the tee-shirts) was simple. I was either working, sleeping, or at the gym. After six months, I received a phone call: Amy was in labor with our son, and it was time to come home. I arrived in Dallas only three days later, travelling constantly by military aircraft. I expected to have missed the main event, but Amy and unborn son had considerately waited for me, and I was able to be present at the birth of our first child. Three weeks later, I was back on the Rock, this time leaving behind not a pregnant wife, but a growing family that I would not see again for another six months.

I never knew what either COBRA or DANE stood for; we passed the time making up colorful suggestions when we weren't working, sleeping, or at the gym. Shemya was a fascinating place then, with multiple tourist attractions: Fifty-Caliber Beach, where the foolish and brave could collect live World War II-vintage ammunition; Shipwreck Beach, where amongst the debris of an old Japanese freighter you could find Coke and 7-Up bottles from the 1940s; numerous fishing holes containing a frighteningly mutated variety of the Dolly Varden trout, which we were warned not only not to eat, but not to even touch, and hundreds of blue foxes from an old, abandoned Russian breeding operation, all with the same genetic defect: a shriveled and useless hind leg. It seemed not to bother them. They hopped on three legs faster than I could run on two.

I also discovered toward the end of my year-long assignment that the drinking water there had been contaminated with diesel fuel. I didn't consider the ramifications until years later.

The remainder of my Air Force career—in Ohio, Colorado, New

Mexico, and many unnamed garden spots around the world—was by turns exciting, stressful, rewarding, frustrating, and uniquely satisfying. Amy and I learned to live together, overlook each other's faults, and adjust to the changes and stresses we encountered. We had a beautiful daughter to go with our handsome son, and were blessed by their ability to survive our mistakes and good intentions. I did fascinating and meaningful work with colleagues I trusted, and I had the opportunity to see and do things that I'll never be able to talk about openly, but which served to solidify the worldview I had held since childhood: the world was hostile and uncaring, and full of malicious intent that could only be challenged and defeated through preparation, analysis, and constant vigilance. During the remainder of my military career, I also continued to serve in operational, research and development, and technology testing assignments that exposed me to a wide variety of environmental hazards and toxic materials. I didn't dwell on it, though. I was doing my job. I was and still am proud to have contributed and honored to have served.

It was a hard way to live, and I didn't have much use for what I called "magical thinking." Magical thinking, by my definition, included wishing, prayer, belief, and hope. One of my father's bits of wisdom that had stuck with me through the years was, "if you wish in one hand and piss in the other, you know which hand is going to fill up first." As vehemently as I tried not to be like my father in any way, that attitude had taken root in me, and it left me a little humorless and intolerant. I was also not much fun at parties.

My ten years in the Air Force were marked by restlessness—I was searching for something that I couldn't find; I didn't even know what I was looking for. I changed jobs more often than normal, and the constant upheaval caused hardships for Amy and my children, even beyond the usual hardships of a military lifestyle. We lived like nomads, moving eight times in those ten years.

I mourned the loss of the fantasy life I imagined would rid me of the feeling of powerlessness and weakness I carried with me. Because of airsickness, sinus infections, and other factors I couldn't control, I would never be a fighter pilot, a test pilot, an astronaut, or the first man on Mars. I knew consciously that it was foolish and childish, but unconsciously I believed those achievements would wash away my shame and self-loathing. I was a military officer, a husband, and the father of two children, but I was also still the preadolescent boy that, paralyzed with fear and dread, had prayed for deliverance and had not received it. I still blamed the God I claimed not to believe in for leaving me alone in the dark as a child, and for denying me the chance to reinvent myself as a strong, fearless, and capable adult.

I wore the trappings of religion like camouflage. Since adolescence, I had had no inward sense of the presence of God or other supernatural phenomena, but I knew better than to be openly scornful. It was unbecoming of an officer and gentleman, or the father of young children and the husband of a good-hearted, loving wife with a strong, sustaining faith. So, I pretended. I taught Sunday school because it looked good on my performance reports, and I helped teach my children the tenets of faith because that's just what one did. I went to church and kept my scorn and criticism to myself (or so I thought; Amy knows me better than anyone, and she was hurt and saddened by my obvious lack of sincere faith). I felt superior; I told myself that a scientist, engineer, and self-proclaimed "rational thinker" knew better than to waste mental energy on medieval superstition, but that if I needed to go along to get along, I would. I was ethical, concerned about doing right and avoiding wrong, and I believed in truth, justice, and the American Way, but I was convinced that there was no otherworldly basis to these beliefs—they were just social convention and the result of evolution acting on social groups. I had it all figured out, and had slapped a coat of paint on my worldview—nothing could penetrate it. God, if He existed, had abandoned and ignored me; I was returning the favor.

Boy, was I dumb.

CAN YOU FEEL ANYTHING WHEN I DO THIS?

June 9, 2011 finally arrived—the day of my deep brain stimulation system implantation. The neurosurgeon had asked us to be at the hospital no later than 5:00 AM. Making a 5:00 AM appointment was not a problem, because I was often still awake then. The night before the implantation had been another sleepless night, but not with apprehension or anxiety, which usually was not the cause anyway. It was just another long night of Parkinson's insomnia, with a touch of added anticipation. Although the likelihood of severe complications from the procedure was very low, I had to assume the worst; so, I had said the things that needed to be said, done everything I could think of to do, and was somewhat at peace.

And then I fell asleep. Parkinson's is like that. Just when you think you have it figured out, it surprises you with something new. So, after eighteen months of incessant insomnia, I was running late for my DBS surgery because I overslept. Amy woke me, and I took a shower with a wonderful disinfectant product called Hibiclens. This was the second of my Hibiclens showers in twelve hours, and was designed to make me less of a threat to myself from infection than I usually am. The primary complication for DBS implantation surgery is post-surgical infection, and my neurosurgeon was taking great pains to avoid that. In general, he had thought through every possible screw-up, unforeseen circumstance, and snafu. I think he might have done this before.

After my leisurely five-minute napalm shower, I threw on some clothes and jumped in the car. We arrived uneventfully at the hospital right at the stroke of 5:00 AM for an abbreviated trip through the admissions office. We had been pre-admitted several days earlier; doing paperwork at three-thirty in the afternoon is much easier than at five in the morning. In rapid sequence we worked our way through surgical admission and then to a holding room for some final medical history and drug interaction discussions.

It became very clear to me that you should never just give yourself over to the system. After a nurse had relieved me of yet another vial of blood, I spoke with another nurse about drug allergies and drug interactions. Those with Parkinson's disease have to be very careful of drug interactions. Some can be fatal, such as the interaction between Demerol and Azilect. I had a very difficult time helping the nurse understand that I wasn't just allergic to Demerol, but that if they gave it to me it would probably kill me. Not that they intended to give me Demerol, of course; however, the longer I talked with her, the more certain I became that as soon as my back was turned they would stab me with a needle full of the stuff. We finally came to an understanding. She told me, "we won't give you Demerol because Azilect has Demerol in it, and you're taking Azilect."

"Not true, but good enough," I said to myself. "I'll just let this one go and take the risk." Amy calls me pedantic, but I think I'm just prudent.

We made our way into the surgical prep area about 5:45 AM, where they started my IV with promises of wondrous treats to come with names I didn't recognize. The surgical nurse told me, "just think of it as a couple of margaritas." That, I could understand. They moved me then to a sheltered corner of the surgical prep area where the first big event of the day would take place—The Shaving. I wasn't overly apprehensive about losing my hair for a short time, but it was still a landmark event for someone who had enjoyed a full head of hair for his entire life. I had no idea what they would uncover. A former college roommate and good friend told Amy, "If you see the number 666 emerging from the hair, try to pretend that it says 999." A Biblical scholar and comedian in one package.

I discovered an interesting phenomenon; when someone has his or her head shaved in the hospital, everyone shows up. Amy, my daughter, the neurosurgeon's entire surgical team, the medical device representative, the nursing staff, the orderlies, and some guy named Walter who wandered in from the hall were all standing around watching as my head was shaved. I wondered who would actually do The Shaving, and was surprised to find that the neurosurgeon himself ran the clippers. Apparently it's all just part of the service.

The Shaving was uneventful, with lots of laughing and joking and comments about the emerging smoothness of my skull, and there were no numerical messages about my role in Biblical prophesy in evidence. The only comment that really stands out came from the neurosurgeon, who apparently moonlights as a standup comedian.

"I've never seen anybody with hair this thick," he said. "You've got hair like a chinchilla."

I didn't have much time to enjoy my new smoothness. Soon after The Shaving was done, Amy and my daughter were escorted to the waiting room and the serious work began. The next major step was installation of the stereotactic frame, which involved local anesthetic, large chunks of machined metal, and some of the biggest screws that I've ever had screwed into my skull. The margarita drugs had started to flow, and my reaction was something like, "OWW!! That hurt…. wha? Hmmm. Look—there's a kitty."

With the contraption now firmly anchored to my skull, they wheeled me down the corridor to the operating theater. I vaguely remember as we were rolling that the anesthesiologist kept telling me, "You don't have to hold your head up off the gurney. Just relax." Yeah, right. Relax.

After a stop for a final CAT scan that I apparently slept through, we arrived at the operating theater. I was awake for the first half of the procedure. From the local anesthetic in my scalp, to the installation of the rest of the stereotactic system, to the distinctive sound of the surgical drill boring nickel-sized holes in the top of my skull, I remember it all. The neurosurgeon told me, "Sorry, this is mashing your nose a little." I think I remember saying, "No biggie; I'm not using it for anything right now anyway."

I remember knowing that they had started to implant the electrodes in my brain, and being satisfied that they were right—it didn't hurt at all. With the benefit of modern pharmaceuticals, I was supremely unconcerned and completely comfortable.

I was also reportedly "pretty chatty" during the first part of the procedure, telling jokes and stories and providing a running commentary on my impressions of the procedure. Perhaps in part to shut me up, they put me to sleep to tunnel the electrical leads under my skin and implant the battery and pulse generator in my chest. The overall procedure was shorter than usual because, according to the neurosurgeon, the electrode placement and the data that they gathered was "just fantastic," and they didn't need to go through the usual neurological testing process to verify placement of the electrodes. That's one of my strongest memories of the whole procedure— the neurosurgeon muttering to himself, "fantastic, just outstanding, this is wonderful, superb…"

I woke up in the recovery room after what seemed like only minutes, with the recovery nurse leaning over me. She smiled and said, "Well, I see you're back." A short time later, Amy came in to visit, and we sat together briefly before they asked her to leave. I spent a long time in recovery, being repeatedly reminded to breathe. The anesthetic they had used depresses respiration, so the nurse kept telling me, "Corey, breathe deeper. Corey, you're not breathing. You need to breathe, Corey." I thought, "Can't you leave me alone? I'm trying to sleep here."

After I left recovery, I headed to the neurological progressive care unit, where I stayed for about thirty-six hours. My family and friends dropped in to wish me well or to make fun of my new look (sometimes both), or to go on walks with me around the corridors. I left the hospital on Friday, just a day and a half after major brain surgery. I could make comments about advances in modern medicine, but I think it's more likely that my insurance company preferred to have me in a lower-cost environment, like my own living room. I had no complaints; I was ready to go home.

I immediately noticed both positive and negative effects from the procedure. Electrode implantation causes some minor damage to the area around the subthalamic nucleus that can result in improvement in Parkinson's symptoms. This effect, called the lesioning effect or the honeymoon period, fades over time, but for two weeks, I could do the neurological testing "finger taps" with my left hand better than any time in the previous five years.

On the negative side, I saw some cognitive changes. There are those who say that I'm always confused; however, I felt that way for several weeks. I thought more slowly, it was difficult to start and finish simple tasks, and I fell asleep unpredictably.

DBS surgery is not a cure, and it's not disease modifying. DBS, like the available drugs, masks the symptoms of PD, but the underlying disease still progresses at the same rate. Having the surgery gave me the gift of time, though. It made time for the biomedical research community to find a cure that can help me and others like me. If there is no cure, it still gave me time to live a fuller, more productive life with the people I love, and vastly improved my quality of life. I was grateful for that time, and I resolved not to waste it.

TRANSITION

In 1994, after nearly ten years on active duty, six permanent change of station (PCS) assignments, a Master's degree courtesy of the US Government, years spent in windowless rooms filled with arcane machinery and documents with colorful cover sheets, and over one million frequent flyer miles on various airlines, Amy and I decided to take advantage of an early-out program offered by the Air Force.

The Department of Defense seems to oscillate between two states: "too much" and "not enough." During the mid-1990s, officers in my career field and year group fell into the "too much" category, and the Air Force was offering money if I would resign and go away. At the time, I was a captain stationed in New Mexico, and I had just been considered and not selected for promotion to major two years early. Amy was weary of the constant moving and searching, my children were old enough that the uprooted lifestyle of the Air Force brat was beginning to take a toll, and I wanted to see how the other ninety-nine percent lived. So we decided to take the offer and separate from the Air Force.

While on active duty, I was involved in a variety of operational, scientific, and engineering activities, almost all of which I still can't discuss. I was exposed to some harsh environments, stresses, and toxins, as many of my colleagues and fellow service members also were, but when I separated, I was as healthy as I had ever been. I was offered the opportunity to be evaluated for service-related disabilities, but I couldn't identify any, with the possible exception of a minor hearing loss. I decided it wasn't worth the effort, and I took my separation paperwork and bid military service farewell almost exactly ten years after entering active duty.

I didn't go far, though—my first civilian job was with a defense contractor that served some of the same organizations I had been aware of while on active duty. It was a familiar environment, and a gentle transition. My leadership and management skills and my technical background were valuable in my new life, and I found I had the ability to project a sense of confidence that I actually didn't feel, but which opened new doors for me. I also found that civilian life, in addition to paying much better than military life, also promoted more quickly, and sometimes for superficial reasons. I rose in the management structure of my new company, and after several years, found myself in the lead of the company's regional office in south Texas, with about 200 employees and a multi-million dollar profit and loss responsibility. I made mistakes, learned from some of them, tried not to repeat them too often, and worked to fill in the huge gaps in my business sense and leadership approach. I constantly felt unqualified for my position, but I was advised by several trusted friends and colleagues to "fake it 'til you make it." Not exactly a winning corporate mission statement, but it got me through the worst times. I learned, faked, and lost sleep, and was successful after a fashion. I was not a naturally talented businessman, but I learned one of the primary secrets to executive success: surround yourself with talented people, give them what they need, and stay out of the way. I was still "looking for it," though, and wanted a new challenge.

A software prototyping project I had supported turned out to have commercial potential, and after a short period of analysis and "walking in the woods" to decide what to do, I became a senior executive in the start-up company formed to commercialize and market the new technology.

I was massively unprepared to be a senior start-up executive, but I had the confidence of youth and inexperience, and I was excited to be a part of a dynamic group of very smart people who had great ideas and wanted to use them to change the world and become rich. This was the late 1990s, at the start of the dotcom boom, and the new conventional wisdom was that you didn't have to show a profit to run a successful business with a lucrative exit strategy. I figured I could make the opportunity work—great ideas, lots of energy, but no actual "P" in the P & L.

Of course, business fundamentals still applied even to dotcoms, and lack of sales eventually whittled away at the company. It was the hardest and most humbling work I've ever done, and I was more talented at some parts of the job than others. Once again, I found I wasn't a naturally talented businessman, but I did have a talent for putting difficult concepts into simple language, and for helping people understand those concepts. I enjoyed teaching and explaining more than deal-making, and I found I was happiest at the front of a room filled with other executives, at a white board or with a set of PowerPoint charts, making the complex simple and the crooked straight.

I began to have periods of severe depression toward the end of my two years in the high-tech start-up world. I blamed unresolved issues from the past and the intense pressure I was under to play a role that didn't fit. The depression became gradually worse and began to noticeably impact my work performance. The downward spiral might have continued to its inevitable conclusion, but circumstance saved me—a large software company showed interested in acquiring the business. They didn't want our customer base (it was laughably small), or our staff (they could have just hired them—we were probably six months from closing the doors anyway). They were interested in our technology—it was truly cutting edge, and one of the reasons we were having trouble selling it was that, in a sixty-minute sales call, we would spend fifty-five minutes explaining the basic concepts and five minutes selling. Potential customers appreciated the education, but wrote no checks.

My depression eased somewhat, but never went away. After the deal was done and all the investors and creditors were paid, there was very little money left for the team (with my cut, I think I bought carpet for the house and a six-pack of good beer), but I had learned a new phrase: founder's stock options. I became an employee of the new company and worked there for the next six years as the value of my options grew, the stock split four times, and a theoretical windfall became real.

I continued to have periods of depression and other odd, seemingly unrelated nuisances and irritations. I noticed that I sometimes would type only with my right hand because my left was aching and stiff. During my many business dinners, I ordered wine less and less often—I didn't enjoy it anymore because I couldn't taste or smell it. On long plane flights, I was restless and uncomfortable and often had to get up and take laps around the plane. And when I was very tired or stressed, my left thumb would twitch. I was working eighty-hour weeks and traveling constantly, so I attributed it to job stress and kept reaching for the gold ring.

I was running out of energy and ideas, though. I became less effective, had more trouble handling company politics and the inevitable jockeying for position and infighting, and I was constantly exhausted. Finally, in the midst of a major merger with another company, I quietly melted down.

Amy could see it coming, although she had no better idea than I did the reason it was really happening. Several months before, she had persuaded me to put our large, expensive executive home on the market. So during the same week that my son, our firstborn, left home to enter college, we also signed a contract to sell our home and I resigned from the company. All we needed was a divorce, a death in the family, and a jail term to round out the list of the topmost stressful events a family can experience, and in typical overachieving style, we did them all simultaneously.

With the temporary reduction in stress that my deconstruction of our entire life brought, I felt free and optimistic again. We moved into an apartment to keep our options open, and I began planning a new type of life for us, free from stress, doing the things that made me happy and fulfilled. My depression and most of my strange afflictions evaporated or lessened, and I told myself, "See? Job stress. Everything will be fine now."

Boy, was I wrong.

RIDING THE LIGHTNING

After my DBS surgery in June of 2011, my incisions healed, my hair grew in true chinchilla style, and I became accustomed to the new lumps, bumps, and ridges on my head and chest. The lesioning effect finally disappeared, but it gave me a preview of how the stimulator might help me and I was eager to turn it on. I had already reduced some drugs and eliminated others, and the device wasn't even working yet. I was sleeping better and the hallucinations had almost disappeared, but in the normal give-and-take of Parkinson's treatment, I was having more tremors and dyskinesia (involuntary wiggling and writhing movements). I didn't miss the squirrels, cats, and phantom people moving around just out of direct sight, though. Life was good, but I was eager for turn-on day.

Exercise is a potent weapon in the battle against PD, and after the surgery I saw again how important it was. When the lesioning effect was at its peak, I decided to stop using the cane I had grown to rely on, and I began to walk for what seemed like several hundred miles every day in an unusual location—the hospital where my DBS surgery was performed. I tried walking in my neighborhood; potentially heatstroke-inducing behavior in south Texas if the walk starts after the sun rises. I tried walking in the mall, too. No. Just no. If I have to explain why, you've never been in a mall.

The hospital was huge, had more corridors than I could walk in a month, and had even more stairs. As an added benefit, no one gave a second glance to the bald guy with the staples in his head walking up and down the stairs and halls with a beautiful and intense woman behind him screaming, "swing your arm, lift your knees, doggone it!" I loved it. I swear.

I had plenty of time while walking to think and talk with Amy about solutions to all the world's problems, and one of our topics of conversation was my cane. I was eager to give it up but I found that it was harder than I expected, and I spent some time examining why. There were the obvious reasons—stability during balance disruptions, help getting in and out of my car (difficult for anyone—I hadn't given up my sports car yet), and added confidence getting up and down stairs. All were completely reasonable physical needs, but not the only reasons the cane was hard to give up, as it turned out.

The physical symptoms of PD can change and worsen over the course of just a few hours, and can ease and improve just as quickly. Some days are better than others, and when I'm doing well, I appreciate comments about how good I look. I know that ninety-nine percent of those comments are honest, sincere, and rooted in kindness and truth. However, I have an unreasonable discomfort with the remaining one percent when I think I can sense an undertone of something else— perhaps an unstated question about how serious this whole thing is anyway, or a level of skepticism about why I'm making such a big deal out of this disease, or a bit of irritation about why I have handicapped license plates on my sports car.

I remember a day when everything seemed to be on a peak—the drugs were working, I had slept well, and I was moving with relative ease. I stopped at a local sporting goods and outdoor outfitters store. Out of habit, I had parked in a handicapped parking spot, knowing that the trip back out could be different than the trip in, and that I could go off at any minute. I left my cane in the car.

When I came out of the store an hour later, I found a penciled note on my windshield.

"You shouldn't park in a handicapped parking spot when you don't need it, a**hole," it said. "Just because you have the tags and it's legal doesn't mean it's right."

I felt a sick sense of indignation. I wanted to find the person who left the note and explain that I wasn't that guy, that I sometimes looked okay but that I really wasn't. I also felt ashamed, as I remembered that there were other people who used handicapped parking spaces who needed them all the time, and were in much worse shape that I was. I resolved then to be more careful about when I used the privilege, but to use it without regret when I needed to.

I discovered, to my surprise, that I carried and used my cane as a kind of explanation, and even an excuse. Why does he limp? Oh, he has a cane— there must be a reason. Why does he fumble with his wallet in the checkout line, drop his change, and take so long? Oh, he has a cane—he's probably sick or injured, and not drunk or clumsy. Why is that young guy parked in the handicapped space? He looks fine—oh, wait, he has a cane. Never mind.

For me, the cane had been not only a physical aid to movement, but also a method for answering questions before they were asked, and a way of opening up conversations about PD on my terms. It was a defense mechanism in the most classic sense, and it showed to me that I wasn't as far along on Dr. Kubler-Ross's five-stage process as I had thought.

I resolved to try to let go of the cane and to trust that the DBS system would do what it was intended to do—reduce the severity of some of my motor symptoms. I also resolved to let go of the one percent and be grateful when I heard, "You really are looking great—I'm glad you're improving."

Turn-on day for my DBS system finally arrived, and was a combination of "rather remarkable" and "no big deal." The neurologist had carefully set my expectations, and I wasn't expecting immediate major changes. As with other elements of my treatment, the neurologist was slow and careful in turning on the stimulator, "titrating up" in electricity just like for new drugs. I was a little disappointed that there was no "oh-my-gosh-I-can-run-jump-and-play-look-at-my-hands-move" moment, but I was happy the thing was working.

The actual programming session didn't take long at all, although I had to stay at the neurologist's office for about two hours after it was done, presumably to see if I would suddenly start picking up radio stations or opening garage doors with my head. The neurologist began by explaining that he would first test the electrical integrity of the leads, and then he would adjust the system to determine how I responded. He was clear that I would leave this first session with the device set at a low level and probably without noticeable effects, and that I would come back in two weeks to have the system tweaked again.

With my expectations properly set (and steam rising from the campfire), he began. I couldn't see the screen of his handheld programming device, so I didn't know what was going to HOLY CRAP, WHAT WAS THAT? I felt a buzzing twitch run down my right arm, and the fingers of my right hand momentarily went into business for themselves. It shut off as abruptly as it started, and I said, "That was strange."

"Yes—that means that the electrode on the left side of your brain is working." For reasons that escape me, the left side of the brain controls motor activity on the right side of the body and vice versa. I started to comment on that fact when my left hand and arm began to twitch and tingle, and my hand became more rigid and immobile than usual. It also was returned to my conscious control quickly, and I had a fleeting thought about the Control Voice at the beginning of the old "Outer Limits" TV show from the early 60s—"There is nothing wrong with your brain. Do not attempt to control your own body. We will control the horizontal, we will control the vertical. We can make you twitch and shake, and if you upset us we will make you sorry."

Things were quiet for a few moments, as the neurologist and the medical device expert discussed next steps in low tones. I was anxiously waiting for the next lightning bolt in some part of my body, but I only felt a few minor tickles and buzzes here and there. I began to relax (always a mistake), and as I tried to settle into the chair and get comfortable, I found that I couldn't. There was no pain or real discomfort, but I couldn't sit still.

"Well, THIS is weird," I said.

Amy, recording the session, said, "What's happening?"

"I can't sit still," I said.

"Are you just trying to get comfortable?"

"No," I replied. "I think I'm trying to dig a hole in the chair."

The neurologist had set the stimulator voltage level, and it caused an immediate and uncontrollable bout of dyskinesia; not painful, just strange. When he reduced the voltage, the dyskinesia evaporated like rain on a Texas street.

Hope is a funny thing—sometimes you have it without knowing it, and just a little extra information changes the picture. I remembered the neurosurgeon's comments about how the "signals were great." That indicated two things: the stimulator was working, and there was no question that I had Parkinson's disease.

You'd think that would be no surprise to me, but I found that I had been holding out some hope that I fell into the fifteen- to twenty-five percent of Parkinson's patients who are misdiagnosed. Diagnosis by neurological exam, medical history, and ruling things out still leaves room for uncertainty, and in a small number of cases, a person treated for Parkinson's for years never actually had the disease. I was still hoping that I would one day wake up without symptoms and find that this had all just been a colossal misunderstanding, even after experiencing classic PD symptoms for years, being diagnosed by five of the best medical professionals in the US, and showing improvement in symptoms after taking levodopa.

I still had hope—for an eventual cure, for a good, productive, happy, and long remainder to my life with people I love, for a manageable progression to this disease, and for long-term effectiveness of DBS. However, I finally had to put away the unreasonable hope that I didn't really have Parkinson's disease.

RECREATION

In the summer of 2006, after I resigned from the company that had made us financially secure, sold my dream house, sent our first born off to college, and tossed the rest of my family into upheaval and uncertainty, I looked around for something else to do. I settled on scuba diving.

My true intent was to take some time off from the stresses and aggravations of the high-tech business world, find out what I really wanted to do, and do a complete reset and reboot of my professional life. Amy and I, after discussing the goals, approach, and available resources, decided I had about a year to decompress and figure it all out. We also discussed the pros and cons of renting either an apartment or a house for that year. We wanted flexibility in case The Plan (version 3.0 now) took us to another city, so we didn't want to buy another house.

We decided to rent an apartment so that our fifteen-year old daughter, who had been ripped up by her roots from her comfortable home, could have the novel experience of apartment living. There are other novel experiences, in retrospect, that would have been better choices: a root canal for her birthday, a sleep-away torture camp, or a new burlap- and barbed-wire wardrobe, for instance. We all survived, but we still call our year in the apartment and the year that followed, "The Lost Years." For such reasons are "good intentions" used as construction materials.

I was hard at work, though. I tried on multiple hats and looked at investment opportunities, alternate careers, and new ways of living. For the first time in my life, I carried a tool kit to work, installing computer and video equipment as an independent consultant with an old friend and former colleague. I hung out a shingle of my own, and did IT security consulting. I considered becoming a real estate agent, a general contractor for home renovations, a franchise restaurant owner, and a safety and training diver in the NASA underwater weightlessness training facility in Houston. The only thing I didn't consider was being an astronaut—that had already been checked off the list.

Between consulting engagements and investment opportunity webinars,

I dived. I was a scuba divemaster and assistant instructor for several of the national scuba certification agencies, so I taught classes at a local dive shop, worked with students who were having difficulty with specific skills, filled and carried scuba tanks, handed out equipment, and lived the life of a dive bum. To give all this activity a veneer of respectability, I developed a business plan for opening a dive shop in an exotic location. Dive shop conventional wisdom says that to make a million dollars in the dive business, you should start with two million dollars. Not so, according to my business plan. It clearly demonstrated how to turn $3.26 million into $1.0 million in just three years. With this bit of due diligence out of the way, I focused in earnest on diving.

I dived almost every day, even if it was just to teach a buoyancy class in the pool or show a problem student how to do a water rescue. My wetsuit never dried out, my skin smelled like chlorine, and my hair was as blonde and brittle as my son's when he was a high school swimmer. I was invited to be the divemaster on a dive trip to Saba, a small island in the Netherlands Antilles, and it was wonderful. I just couldn't figure out how to make being a dive bum support a family of four.

I also began to see some of the old, familiar physical issues return. I had trouble turning the valves on scuba tanks with my left hand when I was filling them, and my left arm and shoulder ached and throbbed constantly. When I was standing in the shallow end of the pool, demonstrating a skill to a group of students or showing them how a piece of equipment worked, I often shivered and shook, even if the water was warm. One of the most obvious issues was apparent on a day I was teaching a group of advanced students underwater navigation skills. As part of the class, each student had to measure the time it took to swim 100 feet underwater in a straight line. As I demonstrated, I was dismayed and embarrassed to discover that I couldn't do it. No matter how carefully I kicked, I curved to the left and ended up twenty-five feet or more from the target at the end of the 100-foot course. The students all got a laugh out of it, but it concerned me. It was obvious that my left leg was much slower and stiffer than my right, and that was something new. I attributed the problems to strain and overuse, and even wondered if with all the diving I had been doing the cause might have been decompression sickness, or "the bends." It didn't get noticeably worse, so I lived with it.

I was no closer to finding the new life I had been seeking and time was passing. I felt like I had jumped from an airplane wearing a parachute harness that either contained a parachute or my dirty laundry, and the only way to find out which was to pull the ripcord, which I had agreed to do within a year. Amy was growing concerned.

"You know, you're probably not going to be able to make a living at diving. Maybe you should start looking for a job."

"I have been looking for a job. I check Monster.com every morning, and I sent a resume out just today," I snapped.

She gave me a familiar look. "I know you wanted something else, but it's been nine months, and now you're just playing. And I also know that you don't really believe you can find the right job by sending out resumes and checking websites."

I fumed, but eventually admitted that she was right. I began looking for a position in my former career field, and hoped that the year-long break would give me a fresh sense of perspective.

I called old colleagues and friends, looking for a way back into the world that I had so unceremoniously abandoned. I found that, regardless of assurances to the contrary, reentry was much more difficult than departure. The economy was starting to falter, positions were filled, people had moved on or retired, and a few held grudges and concerns about my reliability because of my hasty departure from corporate America less than a year before. I found a few entry-level positions, a couple of openings for one hundred percent commission sales jobs, and a few interesting opportunities in San Francisco, Cupertino, or San Jose, the home of the $2 million, 1000-square foot bungalow. I didn't find anything that would work for all of us, though.

Although I was concerned about the return of the pain and stiffness in my arms and legs, I still dived regularly, and volunteered to be the rescue diver for the swimming portion of a local triathlon. It was a simple job—in my wetsuit and with full scuba gear at the ready, I sat in a small fishing boat in the midst of about 100 swimmers and watched and waited. The boat driver was in radio contact with other watchers positioned around the lake, and if any of the racers began to have problems or disappeared below the surface, I would strap in, roll off the boat and be a hero (in theory, anyway).

Fortunately, no one tried to drown, so the boat driver and I struck up a conversation while we scanned the water. He asked me what I did for a living when I wasn't sitting in a boat. I gave him a capsule synopsis, without some of the more colorful elements: Longhorn with a BS in aerospace engineering and an MS in space operations, former Air Force officer, experience with radar, satellite operations and communication, software development and sales, computer security, consulting services, laboratory management experience, business experience in public, private, and start-up companies, currently a dive bum but ready to get back to work. I asked him what he did when he wasn't driving a boat.

"Well, I run a research and development laboratory organization here in town. We do contract-based applied research on communications and electronic systems, and we have a big business in spacecraft subsystem software design. We're trying to build an information security business with commercial and government clients, but we don't have anyone who has the business experience and the interest. I also need some proposal development help, and some general management expertise."

We both sat quietly for a moment, continuing to scan the water. He spoke first.

"Umm, do you think you might like to come in for an interview?"

"I think that would be great," I said. "Since almost every experience I've had in my life up to this point has prepared me for this conversation, it would be ungrateful not to."

I talked with him and his team several times over the next two months, and they agreed to let me work with them. I wasn't a perfect fit; these people were as good or better than every scary-smart scientist or engineer I had ever met, and I had let my hardcore engineering skills atrophy in favor of developing business skills. They recognized they weren't hiring me for my 1980s and 1990s-vintage engineering expertise, but for a combination of engineering outlook and business experience. They were kind enough never to use the phrase, "a mile wide and an inch deep" in my presence.

I started work there, and as expected, the learning curve was steep. As the leader and manager of people smarter and more technically current than myself, I was expected to keep up, and to also find paying work of my own I could do (no one likes a freeloader). I had learned a few tricks along the way, though.

In meetings during the first few months, I struggled to come up to speed quickly. I took copious notes, and when anyone asked my opinion or wanted direction, I cultivated the thoughtful look and the chin-stroke, and said, "Well, what are your recommendations? Surely you must know what you'd like to see happen here?" I usually escaped unscathed, and I could then spend all evening on the Internet answering the same question over and over again in different technical areas: "What in the world does THIS mean?"

I loved the work, I respected and admired the people I worked with, and I found that the man I had met unexpectedly in a boat on a lake was the best boss I had ever had—he was not only a gifted engineer, but he was a good businessman and a genuinely good person, and he became a friend as well as a colleague. My job stresses were normal and manageable, especially after having had experience in the Roman arena of commercial high-tech, and I felt that, at long last, I had finally found home. I intended to finish my professional career there. As it turned out, I did.

One by one, the physical symptoms and collection of strange difficulties that had plagued me for almost two decades returned. This time, I couldn't ignore them or blame job stress. I had no choice but to find out why this was happening.

I'LL HAVE TWENTY-TWO HELICOPTERS AND A FUDGSICLE

My neurologist activated my DBS system in July of 2011. I had a programming session about every two weeks for several months, and the benefits of DBS soon became clear. I had more consistent symptom control, and my medication side effects were much more manageable. I also had an electronic device embedded in my body, which I thought was pretty cool.

Although my neurologist instructed me in strong terms not to play with the device, I felt it was only prudent to understand how it worked, and to know how to turn it on and off if I needed to. Perhaps I should have I should have read the FULL manual before I began claiming that my stimulator battery was malfunctioning, and begin hauling medical device representatives, neurosurgeons and neurologists, and people off the street into a room to discuss what was wrong with the darned thing. When, oh when will I ever learn to listen to my wife?

Amy said, "It's probably just the batteries in the patient programmer, don't you think?"

I didn't think—that was my first problem. My second problem was that I didn't listen to Amy.

"Naaaah, can't be. I remember clearly that someone at some point said something about a percentage level, related to something that I don't remember but that I'm convinced has to do with the stimulator battery. That makes sense, doesn't it?"

It didn't. The neurologist placed me under strict orders to think about topics other than my stimulator, and to give the "Electro Boy" fascination a rest. How unfair, I thought. What's the fun of having a new electronic device that's actually inside my brain if I couldn't have a little fun with it now and then? In retrospect, perhaps I had the wrong attitude about the whole situation. My credibility suffered, and I pouted that I was being unfairly blamed for a natural response, especially for someone who had a passion for electronics. I consoled myself by playing with my fleet of helicopters.

Which brings me to a slightly more serious subject, although at the time it didn't seem all that serious. Over a period of about eighteen months, I developed an interest in model helicopters. They were fascinating—they're complex little devices, you can break them and put them back together endlessly, and with practice you can fly them around the room and chase the cat with them. For someone with both aeronautical and electronic interests, they are an almost perfect diversion.

You'd think that one or two would be enough to satisfy nearly anyone. Not so, particularly someone with compulsive behavior side effects from Parkinson's medications. It was slow and insidious, like many things associated with Parkinson's disease, but over a year and a half I developed quite a fleet of model helicopters. At one point I had twenty-two of them. In the clear light of retrospection, even I can see how bizarre that was. It's not unusual behavior for someone with PD taking a dopamine agonist drugs, however. As matter of fact it's benign given the possible spectrum of behaviors.

Compulsive behavior caused by dopamine agonists can include compulsive gambling, hypersexual behavior, compulsive shopping (for helicopters, for instance, or home electronics, or home automation equipment, or Fudgsicles, just to name a few random possibilities), or an obsessive focus on almost any activity or object. The behavior is a medication side effect, but the consequences are real and can cause upheaval, relationship damage, and financial ruin for the unwary. Like the physical symptoms that I was able to explain away, I was able to justify my focus on model helicopters as a healthy way to replace other interests that I had lost: scuba diving, sports, running, skiing, and most other physical activities. After all, everyone needs a hobby, right?

My compulsive behavior was relatively easy to control, and the impacts were minor (although I did have a few pounds to lose from all those Fudgsicles). The realization that I was behaving compulsively, however, opened up a new set of possibilities to consider. They were hard to contemplate, but they are a part of Parkinson's disease and can't be ignored.

In addition to the motor and autonomic nervous system symptoms associated with PD, there is a spectrum of potential cognitive impacts. They range from minor short-term memory disruption to severe dementia almost as profound as Alzheimer's disease. According to the medical literature, nearly every Parkinson's patient experiences some cognitive issues, even if they are mild and not significantly more noticeable than the usual effects of aging.

My family and friends had noticed initial indications of something called "executive dysfunction" in me. Although it sounds like a bad quote from a Dilbert cartoon, it's related to the ability to multitask, to think abstractly, to remember and apply facts, and to interpret motivations and read situations effectively.

I had trouble remembering new facts, and regularly missed appointments even though I kept a calendar on my phone. My job required me to juggle the details of dozens of complex technical projects; if I had enough time I could retrieve the information I needed from my failing brain, but there was never enough time. I became more and more ineffective at business development and customer relationships; my occasional stammering, difficulty remembering details, and slowness in switching subjects left me a half-step behind, and I avoided activities that were critical to my job performance.

My DBS system made my motor symptoms more manageable, and exercise and physical therapy improved my movement problems. My autonomic nervous system irregularities could be improved by a combination of lifestyle changes, medications, and simple tolerance. However, the combination of physical and newly emerging cognitive problems caused significant disability.

So finally, in August 2011, after twenty-seven years of a satisfying and varied professional life as a military officer, an executive in public, private and start-up companies, and a leader and manager in the nonprofit research and development world, Amy and I decided that it was time for me to retire. I began disability leave from work, and given the nature of this disease, I don't anticipate returning to my professional career. It was the hardest decision of many hard decisions we've made since I was diagnosed, but it was the right one.

I made the choice in the initial stages of the disease to be aggressive in addressing the symptoms. Some doctors and PWPs will counsel "saving some for later." For instance, young-onset patients like me often are counseled to avoid a drug called carbidopa-levodopa for as long as possible, because long-term exposure usually has the side effect of significant disability from dyskinesia. However, without it, I was always "off" (the term a PWP uses to describe a period when the symptoms are at their peak, and when they're not getting much or any relief from the treatments). I decided to take the risk of debilitation from dyskinesia later for the reward of better function and enhanced quality of life now, and I began taking carbidopa-levodopa almost immediately. The same rationale applied to my decision to have DBS surgery, and to an extent, to my decision to retire from professional life. I decided to do everything I could to maximize quality of life now, and to leave the future to medical research and good fortune.

When I retired, the changes in me were sometimes less apparent during the day. In particular, some of the changes Amy saw only she was able to recognize, because no one knows me as well as she does. She was there when I got out of bed in the morning, and saw what I was like before my morning handful of pills. She saw me stumble and trip at night when I had had an exhausting day, and meds and DBS together couldn't mask my symptoms. She saw me struggle to find words, hesitate, and lose track of a conversation. And she saw the radical increase in all my symptoms from simple, everyday work stress. She knew better than anyone that it was time to let go, and she helped me to see it, too.

Everyone approaching middle age begins to have physical and cognitive problems, some worse than others. Taken in isolation, each of the challenges I was managing was inconsequential. But, when coupled with other inconsequential problems that were fundamentally out of character for me, a pattern began to develop. I could tell there was something changing. It was slow and hard to notice—one day was not significantly different than the next. But one week was slightly different from the next, one month was noticeably different the next, and last year was significantly different from this year. I could deny it or I could acknowledge it, fight it, and live with it where I couldn't fight it. I'd had enough denial.

DO NOT GO GENTLE…

In the first several months after I retired, I had trouble wrapping my head around the concept that the change was real and permanent, barring an act of God or a miraculous cure. Although I could find plenty to occupy my time, I felt like I was playing hooky from school, and I couldn't shake the feeling that my e-mail box at work needed attention. There must be some sort of natural law related to conservation of e-mail, however, because my personal email stepped into the gap.

I discovered that while I had been focusing on work in the last few years, I had seriously neglected my handy-man responsibilities around the house. I was surprised and dismayed to find out that my sprinkler system didn't work very well and that Amy had known it for years. So, without considering the limitations imposed by chronic illness and recent surgery, I pitched into the project of repairing the sprinkler system. I didn't think too deeply about the fact that there was a terrible drought in progress in south Texas, with lawn watering restricted to no more than once per week. Regardless of how well the sprinkler system worked, the yard was going to be dead anyway, but that seemed beside the point.

That summer was among the hottest in Texas history, also—a perfect time to spend hours in the sun doing manual labor that I had been completely unaccustomed to doing in recent years. The good thing about working on a sprinkler system is that you can pretend to be examining the function of the sprinkler heads and adjusting the spray pattern with a little screwdriver, when you're actually letting the sprinkler spray you in the face and praying for a cloud to come by so that you don't die from heat stroke.

Although I tried not to dwell on it, I was still finding new ways that Parkinson's disease intruded on activities I used to take for granted. Most people probably know that a sprinkler system is underground. I didn't realize that "underground" is a significant journey for someone with PD. It takes quite a while to get there, and it takes even longer to get back after you've spent some time there. Digging up sprinkler heads and valves is challenge for anyone when the Texas sun is roughly thirty feet away and the temperature in the shade is like a summer day on Venus; PD only adds additional fun.

It's also advisable to sit on the ground while working; bending over becomes painful, and you end up with a sunburn that's hard to explain. For someone with Parkinson's, blood pressure variations from changing posture (postural hypotension) can turn the act of standing up into a quick trip back to the ground and a brief nap. A little prior planning was in order.

I hadn't done much of this kind of work in the recent past, and I had to make a few accommodations. Gravity is helpful on the way down, as long as you don't make the trip so quickly that the impact causes discomfort. However, climbing out of the gravity well again was an entirely different experience than I remembered from just a few years ago. I understood how a box turtle must feel, lying on his back, waving his claws in the air and slowly roasting on a Texas highway.

There's a way to solve any problem, though, even mobility problems caused by Parkinson's disease. I started carrying a small chair with me so the up-and-down journey was not quite as disconcerting. To combat the heat, I soaked my Harley-Davidson do-rag with water from the hose, draped it over my nearly bald head, and covered it with a baseball cap to protect my freshly healed DBS scars. I thought I was clever, and maybe even a little bit cool because I was wearing Harley logoware, until I saw my neighbor laughing and shaking his head. Maybe it's just that I was wearing the wrong color do-rag. I had no idea the neighborhood was Crip instead of Blood.

Everything takes longer with PD, so I had plenty of time to think as I spent thirty minutes screwing six screws into a sprinkler system valve cover, and that was with an electric screwdriver. Why was it important to me to do these things? Since having DBS surgery, I had risked heatstroke, rattlesnakes, Gila monsters, and fatal sunburn while working on the sprinklers, as well as Amy's displeasure for falling through the bedroom ceiling while working in the attic pulling Ethernet cable. Why?

The fact of my recent retirement provided a partial answer. Under different circumstances, I might have had another fifteen to twenty years of useful work left to me, doing important and valuable work that would have continued to give me a sense of fulfillment, mission, and purpose. I grieved for that lost potential, and I took on projects as a way to continue to have a sense of value and purpose, even if my capacity was not what it used to be. I enjoyed my ability to make things work, to fix broken machinery, and to solve problems. Occasionally those problems were of my own making, but if you're going to dig yourself into a hole, it's helpful to be able to dig out again. Although it took ten times longer than in my pre-PD days, fixing the sprinkler system reminded me that I still had the capacity to solve problems and to accomplish difficult tasks, even if the definition of "difficult" had changed.

Another equally important answer to the question, "why do I do these things?" was that it was a way to *fight back*. Life with PD is a daily battle: against exhaustion, drug side effects, nausea, stiffness, slowness, tremor, pain, and all of the other baggage this unwelcome visitor brings. I tend to think in military metaphors, and I once described Parkinson's disease as a long battle against overwhelming odds from a succession of fallback positions. There are many ways to feel like a loser in this situation, but there are just as many ways to feel like a winner. One of those ways is by simply not giving in. I was not successful every day, but every day brought another opportunity. I fixed the sprinkler system, pulled Ethernet cable, expanded the home automation system, and even flew those helicopters as a way to say to Parkinson's, "Today, I win. Tomorrow may be different, but just for today, the battle goes to me." That was worth aching muscles, minor sunburn, blisters, losing ten screws for every one I got into the right place, and even the occasional need to patch a hole in the ceiling. PD may be an overwhelming, unstoppable adversary, but I resolved to make sure it knew it was in a fight.

RATIONALIZATION

I still remember the smell—cigarette smoke, Old Spice aftershave, sweat, and a peculiar sour odor I would later recognize as fear. I was six years old, and when I sat in my father's police cruiser, I always got dizzy and sick to my stomach because of the smell.

My father was already a captain in the police department when I was born. I knew very little about his role as police officer as I was growing up; he left in the morning before I got out of bed, and I didn't see him again until shortly before bedtime, when he would come home smelling like his police cruiser, place his service weapon in the cabinet above the refrigerator, and sit down to dinner.

I lived in awe and fear of my father. Our family used to say that my dad could "shout with his eyes." He rarely had to raise his voice to get our attention. When he was happy, he was magnanimous and jovial, witty and funny, everyone's friend. But when he was not, you could tell by the storm clouds in his eyes.

As a police officer, my father used fear and intimidation as behavior management tools. He told stories at the dinner table about keeping criminals and prisoners in line by intimidating them with the threat of violence without actually needing to use violence. He prided himself on never having had to draw his service weapon, except the one time that he drew his 1911 pistol to repeatedly apply it to an unruly prisoner's head in the elevator on the way to the booking room. The pistol broke, he said, and I presume the prisoner's skull did as well. That was unusual for Dad, though. He could apply the concept of deterrence just as effectively as the US government did to control Soviet aggression during the Cold War.

My father was not typically physically violent, but he understood the application of force and the use of mental and emotional intimidation to control other people. He was proud of his ability to use the power of his personality to get what he needed and wanted from others, including his wife and children. My dad scared me, but like any six-year-old boy, I longed to be like him. After all, he obviously wasn't afraid of anything; he made other people afraid, and that gave him a power that I craved. When I was older, I overheard him tell my brother, "Make sure they never know just how far you're willing to go. Keep them wondering how bad you might hurt them, and they'll comply." I believed him completely; I had seen it.

A mythology grew around my father as I grew older. He was larger than life. His wife and children willingly assumed the burden of recounting the family history, and he was usually the central figure in that history. The victors write history, and my father always made sure he was the victor.

"Remember the time that Dad ran out of gas, and all the rest of us were too afraid to say anything? Corey was too young to know better, and he kept asking, 'Dad, why are we stopping? Why are we stopping, Dad? Are we there? This doesn't look like the campground. Are we camping here?' We had to pin him down in the back seat and hold our hands over his mouth to keep him from making Dad mad. Wasn't that funny?"

"Remember when Kathy snapped Dad on the butt with the dish towel, and he told her not to do it again or she would be sorry? She did it again, and he took the dishtowel away from her and began whipping her with it. She ran out the front door, and he chased her down the block for nearly half a mile whipping her while she screamed. Wasn't that funny?"

"Remember when Mom told us about the time when they were newlyweds and Dad said she should never hit him, because she wouldn't like what would happen in return? Mom didn't think he was serious, and so she playfully slapped him once, and he slapped her back nearly hard enough to knock her out. Dad sure is a man of his word, isn't he?"

"Remember when Dad told Ken that he was the laziest tennis player he had ever seen, and if he wasn't going to try harder to live up to his potential, Dad wouldn't waste his time coming to see him play? Dad was tough, but he just wanted us to do our best."

We told these stories proudly, adding our family interpretation of each event just as we had been taught. Only when we began to tell these stories together after my parents died in late 2000, or when I told them to people outside the family, did a different interpretation begin to emerge.

Some of the proudest stories in our family mythology concern my father's role in a national crisis during the early 1960s. Although he was not actually present at the Kennedy assassination, he played an integral role in press relations in the following days, and he testified before the Warren Commission concerning his and the police department's activities during the subsequent investigation. Although I was too young to remember the actual event, I do remember the stories.

"When Kennedy was assassinated in Dallas, Dad was the police chief's right-hand man with the press. He worked for three days straight, doing almost all the press conferences because the chief disliked talking to the press. He didn't come home for almost a week. He really worked hard for the things he believed in."

"After Oswald killed Officer Tippit, Dad helped manage the fund of donations for his family. When the fund became bigger than anyone expected, and the Chief wanted to put some of the money in the Police Widows and Orphans Fund, Dad argued with him and finally told him, 'That money belongs to Mrs. Tippit. If you do this, my first stop will be at the personnel office where I will resign. My second stop will be the Dallas Morning News editorial office, where I will tell them everything.' Dad was really able to put it all on the line for the things he believed, wasn't he?"

I had the rare opportunity of seeing a YouTube video of one of my father's press conferences during the crisis, and I was amazed at what I saw. He was calm, competent, and in charge, and it made me unwillingly proud to see him. He was at the focus of the derision and criticism of the entire world for a time, and he was masterful.

Certainly, press relations between police departments and the press have changed in the last fifty years, and are now much more open. But, I also recognized what I saw in my father's eyes. I saw the storm clouds there, and I knew how angry he was.

He was angry that the reporters would dare to second-guess the department's actions during the crisis, and was personally offended by their insinuations that the department was incompetent. He was angry at having to justify the actions of men who he considered to be heroes, and I remember more than once in later years that he said, "The whole world thought that we were Keystone cops. They just didn't get it." And, I also think he was angry that the power of his personality and his ability to intimidate and coerce were not effective. He couldn't control perceptions as much as he wanted, and it enraged him.

He could control his own emotions, though. He was calm, cool, and professional, and didn't overtly display the rage I had learned to recognize in his eyes. Fifty years after the event and ten years after his death, I felt a chill as I watched that video. I thought, "Don't they know how mad they're making him? Don't they know what could happen?" And I realized, no, they didn't. You had to be family to know.

The Kennedy assassination became a subject that we never discussed at home. Dad would not answer questions about it from us, and he scoffed at conspiracy theories and accusations of involvement of the department, the FBI, and the Secret Service in the assassination. He had about as much use for alternative theories of the assassination as he did for the Beatles or for long hair.

Although I believe that doing the right thing was important to my father, it was clear that appearing to do the right thing was at least as important. "Avoiding even the appearance of impropriety" was a phrase that I heard repeatedly as I grew up with my father. His message clearly was that, regardless of what might actually have happened, appearing to be without reproach was ultimately the most important thing in any situation.

My father was a mix of good and bad, and I suspect he knew it. He was respected and loved by many of his colleagues, who spoke glowingly of the positive influence he had had on their lives, and how much of a role model he had been. I couldn't count the number of people who came to me at his memorial service to tell me stories about how honorable, noble, and selfless he was. I smiled and nodded, thinking, "You just didn't know him." It didn't occur to me until later that perhaps they knew things about him that I didn't know or couldn't see.

Dad craved that kind of adulation, but he also had his own demons. I had seen him struggle with anxiety and panic attacks since I was old enough to observe and understand. There was always an alternate explanation: throat spasms that caused him to choke and wheeze, stomach problems, job stress, heart disease. Any explanation was better than the truth, because the truth wasn't a part of the carefully crafted public persona he had built. I think the truth was that he was haunted by many of the things he had done, and he couldn't admit it even to himself.

"Mother is the name for God in the lips and eyes of little children," according to the novelist William Thackeray. If that's true, I think it's equally true that Father is the voice and face of God. For most children, the first view they have of God is their own father. I was afraid of mine, and later revolted by him, and then ashamed and deeply disappointed in him. In the end, the fiction he created and maintained at all costs was more important to him than I was, and I rejected everything he taught and claimed, regardless of its truth or value. And in that mix, I rejected the possibility that God might exist, and then built rational reasons for holding that view. My own truth, though, is that the rejection came first and the reasons came later.

My reasons for rejecting even the concept of God were specific and well developed. A treasured family friend once asked me, "What has having PD done to your theology?" His innocent, well-intentioned question was the beginning of several years of email correspondence and personal visits, during which I laid out the carefully reasoned basis for my lack of belief. I argued, pointed out inconsistencies of fact in the Bible, used analogy and metaphor, applied inductive and deductive logic, and expounded learnedly about biology, physics, mathematics, and philosophy. I endlessly defined and redefined terms, talked about the scientific method, waxed poetically about the value of uncertainty and the quest for truth and knowledge, and quoted everyone from Bertrand Russell to Carl Sagan. I was earnest and sincere, and I convinced myself many times over. However, I never admitted or recognized that all this reasoning didn't come first—the rejection did. Regardless of the validity of the arguments, they were built on sand. I didn't reject God because reason led me there. I rejected God for emotional, non-rational reasons, and then used reason to help me stay there. It was time to start over, and build up from the foundation again.

THE ELECTRIC JITTERBUG

About six months after the DBS system was implanted, I began experiencing a recurrence of the "on-off" phenomenon—fluctuations in my physical symptoms due to changes in medication levels. One of the reasons for using DBS was to help smooth out those variations, but I had started to crash again after a medication dose wore off. Two or three times a day, I suddenly and unpredictably became stiff, slow and shaky, and I stayed that way until the next dose of medication took effect. I discussed the problem with my neurologist, and he suggested that increasing the DBS voltage level should help. By then this was familiar territory, so I was unfazed by the normal tickles, buzzes, and jolts I felt as he tested the system. He settled on a new stimulation level, and since I seemed to tolerate it well, he suggested I have lunch and come back in an hour or so.

As I left the office and headed toward my car, I started to feel... well, I don't know how to describe it. "Twitchy" might be the right word, but it really doesn't do the feeling justice. I began having trouble walking when I was about 100 feet from the car, and by the time I unlocked the door I was having trouble standing. My entire body was completely uncontrollable, with jerky, thrashing movements that were worsening by the minute.

I had a completely inappropriate response to the situation—I began to laugh. I've been a Monty Python fan for years, and I imagined suddenly having become a charter member of "The Ministry of Silly Walks." I got in the car, telling myself, "Well, this is kind of funny, but I need to calm down. I'm hungry, and I can't drive like this." I decided that through sheer force of will, I could stop thrashing so I could have lunch.

My force of will had no effect. The dyskinesia steadily worsened, and I grew concerned. The uncontrolled movement had become violent, and the first time I punched myself in the face I decided I had had enough. I tried to cross my arms and hold my hands still, but that wasn't working either. My legs were kicking and thrashing, and my arms were beating against the steering wheel, the gearshift, the rear view mirror, and my own face and body. It took me ten minutes to get back into the doctor's office.

I looked like a rag doll in a high wind, and I caused quite a stir in the waiting room. The doctor's assistant knew immediately what had happened, and he hustled me back to an examination room. It didn't take long to readjust the stimulation level and stop the dyskinesia, and this time I waited in the doctor's office until we were both sure it was over. Afterwards, I was no worse for wear other than bruises on my arms and legs, a couple of sore spots on my face, and an all-over body soreness from getting a week's worth of exercise in fifteen minutes. It was a frightening experience, but I think the most frightening thing about it was my realization that for many Parkinson's patients, this is an everyday experience that goes on for years, as a side effect of long-term exposure to levodopa. It's another reason that research into the cause of PD is important, so we can stop using treatments that end up being worse than the disease itself.

EXPLORATION

Discovering that I had a degenerative, incurable disease threw a harsh light on my values, prejudices, and beliefs, both conscious and unconscious. It shook my confidence and caused me to question my basic sense of self. And, it created a desire for self-assessment and evaluation: "What have I done with my life? What do I have left to do? How long do I have? What should I do with my time? What do I really believe? Why am I here?"

In other words, it made me a particularly irritating conversational partner, and I drove away a fair number of people for a while by being unable to have a normal conversation. I tended to stifle friendly interchange.

"Hey, it's good to see you! How have you been? How's your family?"

"I'm fine, they're fine. How can an omniscient, omnipotent, omnibenevolent God exist when evil and pain are present in the world?"

"Umm, well... yeah. You take care, okay?"

I received an email from my father-in-law's old Army buddy and dear family friend who had recently retired from a long career as an engineer and corporate executive, and who was now a missionary in Mozambique. We had a surprising number of things in common, and we started an email correspondence that lasted for over a year. He was able to overlook the fact that I was a Texas Longhorn, and I overlooked his unfortunate affiliation with Texas A&M University, and although we were different in age and experience we shared life stories and kept up with developments in each other's lives. I learned that his wife and son had Huntington's disease, and that his family was working through the consequences and implications. His experiences helped me to understand the fears Amy had in her role as a caregiver, and my journey with Parkinson's gave him insight into the fears and challenges his wife and son were facing.

We also shared views on spirituality and the role of religion in our lives. Since I knew he was a missionary, I expected the hard sell—I was familiar with evangelical fervor from my encounter with the major in pilot training and with others since then, and I considered myself to be well armed and impervious. I explicitly (and arrogantly) laid out the ground rules: we could discuss whatever he wanted to along those lines, but I had heard it all before, and he had nothing new under the sun to offer me. I wasn't quite that terse and offensive, but I was clear that I thought the ground was well plowed, and I had a counter-argument to everything he might say to persuade me to his viewpoint. I half-expected him to say, "Well, all right then," and never to hear from him again.

His response surprised me, though. "Fair enough," he said. "I don't claim to have a lock on the truth, but I suspect you don't, either." His sincere attitude was that perhaps we both had things to teach, and he repeatedly proved his sincerity by listening as much as he talked. I gave him things to think about and he returned the favor, and we had a lively but largely academic exchange of ideas. I trotted out my list of unanswerable questions and showstoppers, and as usual I was prepared to refuse to consider arguments that weren't supported by my definition of evidence. I was prepared to resist so strongly that I almost fell over when he didn't push. Instead, he told me stories.

He told me about his life and experiences in Africa. He told me about how difficult it was for him to be a man of faith in the business world. He told me about his triumphs and successes, and about his failures and regrets. He told me what it was like for him to be both a rational, hardheaded engineer and a Christian, and how he thought the two could coexist. He told me about himself; he offered me no universal truths, proofs, or incontrovertible evidence. Little by little, he just told me his story. He was limited by the medium of email, but he didn't preach and he didn't push.

When I was growing up, I was immersed in church life. My mother and father met in the church choir. We were Methodists, and we attended church every Sunday. I remember being baptized, and my first spanking was the result of misbehavior in church. I even sang in my grandparents' church when I was about five. My rendition of "Bless This House" made them proud, but even then there was clearly no recording contract in my future.

When we moved to DC, the whole family seemed to drift away from spiritual life. My father insisted that we keep up appearances, but I had already begun to resist by the time the abuse began. I have no significant memories of church, no recognition of God's presence in my life, and no sense of external moral guidance from the time I was seven years old until well after I was married. I began with a vague sense of embarrassment at the concept of God that evolved into an unconscious rejection when the abuse was ongoing, and became a conscious, total rejection of God, religion, spirituality, and all the associated trappings as a teen and young adult.

How did I see the world? I had never tried to summarize my worldview until my friend asked the question, and I spent some of my sleepless nights trying to answer that question for myself. I called myself a scientific rationalist, and I defined that label through these contentions:

– Belief in anything without accompanying evidence is indefensible, and "evidence" has a very rigorous definition. It includes things that can be independently examined by other people, but not personal, inward experiences and perceptions.

– The best toolset we have for evaluating evidence is the scientific method. It's not infallible, because people are not infallible, but as a principle of thought and behavior it has power.

– There must be a foundation of evidence available to be tested and re-evaluated for all our beliefs, but it's not necessary to retest that evidence constantly. There's uncertainty, potential for error, misperception and misinterpretation of observations, and other risks and pitfalls, but that's unavoidable.

– The universe operates according to natural principles that may not be completely known, but which are potentially knowable. As time goes on, we have consistently discovered more about those natural principles and pushed back the boundaries of ignorance, and it appears we may eventually understand the fundamentals of the principles on which our existence is based. The discovery process is awe-inspiring and exciting, but there's no scientific evidence that it's mediated or managed by supernatural forces.

–¬ Science, although flawed, is a fundamentally sound way of understanding our world and our place in it. Skeptical inquiry into root causes, explanations, foundations, and reasons for the things we see and experience is valuable.

– There is no credible scientific evidence of supernatural actors or effects in the world. The things that lead people to belief in supernatural forces are more easily explained by known or as-yet undiscovered natural causes. Lack of explanation is due to current gaps in knowledge, incomplete observation, or errors in perception or evaluation.

– Like the scientific method, the principle called Occam's Razor is useful for evaluating causes and evidence. It's not a belief system, it's just a tool in what Carl Sagan called "the universal baloney detector toolkit."

As a personal philosophy it's a little cold and dry, but it appealed to my need for order and logic and served to protect me from the unexplainable elements of life. When I dug deeper, though, I discovered attitudes that were not based on coldly logical rationality, but which were instead messy and inconvenient:

– I had a deep desire to believe that existence had meaning other than the meaning we create for ourselves. I didn't know where it came from, but if I was truthful, I had to admit it was there. I had a "God-shaped hole" in my being.

– If God existed, I was at a loss to understand His nature. He had ignored me when I needed Him most, and allowed me to suffer for no reason I could see. To be blunt, I couldn't believe in God, because if he existed, I hated Him.

– I was embarrassed by my desire for a higher purpose, and I believed that it was just a symptom of unresolved damage from my childhood history of abuse and my search for a father I could trust. It was wish fulfillment at its worst, and it was a sign of the weakness and powerlessness I dreaded so strongly.

– I rejected belief in the unexplainable. I had a sincere love for scientific, rational thought, and I thought that accepting non-rational beliefs was a slippery slope to irrationality, dogmatism, and small-mindedness.

– I believed that science and faith really were at odds, and if I had to choose, I preferred science. Faith and trust just got me into trouble, and I had made terrible mistakes in believing and trusting the wrong things. It was safer to withhold judgment in an environment of uncertainty, even one that dealt with attitudes, emotions, and values rather than facts.

My missionary friend and I corresponded about other things, but we always came back to this subject. I followed my normal pattern of asking hard questions, not to seek answers but to prove a point. He didn't rise to the bait, though. He said, "That's an interesting question; I don't know the answer" as often as he said anything else, but wasn't disturbed or embarrassed by his lack of refutations. He just kept telling me stories of his life.

I was unmoved, secure in my fortress of rationality and reason, sure I had it all figured out and afraid that I was right. I figured that the only path forward was through answers I could accept to those unanswerable, academic questions, and I both feared and longed for those answers.

I received an email from him telling me that his wife's Huntington's disease had progressed to the point that they needed to return home to Texas, probably for good. He said they both would miss the people and their work together in Mozambique, but that he looked forward to meeting me. I looked forward to it, also—even through the limited forum of email, I had grown to like and respect him, and I was eager to meet him in person. It would be the beginning of a profoundly impactful friendship and a life-changing experience for both of us.

THINGS FALL APART...

I'm sure that William Butler Yeats was not writing about my home automation system, but his poem was uncomfortably appropriate. I had discovered that building a system of computer-controlled lighting and other home technologies was even more fun than flying model helicopters; not only could I chase the cat, but I could open the door as he ran in feline panic across the front hallway, and then lock the door behind him and watch him with the security cameras as he stalked around the yard, looking for a way back in. This is a hypothetical example; I haven't actually done it. I'm just pointing out that it's possible.

However, when a home automation system goes bad, it's much worse than just picking up a few parts off the floor and patching a small hole in the wall. After spending months of sleepless nights watching the shadows, listening to the whispers, and building a smart house, I found myself embroiled in a home automation Chernobyl. Without realizing it, I had built a house of electronic cards, and it only took one simple failure for almost all of it to come tumbling down.

I first became interested in home automation after a discussion with a colleague at work. His description was fascinating, and it had all the right elements to capture my attention: cool electronic gadgets to buy, the need to take things apart and put them back together again, a reason to buy new tools, and the remote possibility of a workable system when I was finished. He sealed the deal for me when he showed me his home system from his office computer and told me that if he wanted to, he could turn the lights on in his master bathroom from where we sat. If you feel the need to ask why this is necessary, I can't help you.

I was particularly prone to influence, since I had realized that my scuba diving days were over and I was in search of a gadget-filled, equipment-intensive new hobby that didn't place my own life or someone else's at excessive risk. Coincidentally, we had this discussion just a few months after I had started taking a dopamine agonist, so without knowing it, I was just itching to become obsessively involved with some new activity. Life isn't all

Fudgsicles and helicopters.

The next eighteen months were filled with online shopping trips, replacing perfectly functional light switches, power outlets, and junction boxes with computer-controlled equivalents at ten times the price, and vastly over-engineering my home network just for fun. I was both proud and ashamed of the fact that I had as many terabytes of data storage as I had pairs of Vibram Five-Finger shoes (another brief but intense obsession).

Then came the control software, the security cameras (eight of them, to keep tabs on the cat), the electronic door locks, the touchscreen control panel, the energy management system, the motion sensors, and the computer-controlled landscape lighting and garage door. My friend had warned me that this would happen. I wish I could blame it all on the medication, but it might have happened anyway.

I eventually gained some knowledge and expertise, but I never took the time to go back and correct the mistakes I made during the early installations. So, when the lights in the kitchen began to inexplicably flash whenever we opened or closed the garage door, when any light in any location in the house turned on or off, or when I locked the doors at night, I begin to suspect something was wrong.

Any competent network engineer can quote the mantra of network troubleshooting: "check the physical layer first." Except for that bit of wisdom, you never really know where to start; the hardware guys always blame the software, the software guys blame the hardware, and everybody claims, "… it must be a distant end problem." I had no one to blame but myself, since I was both the hardware guy and the software guy, and the most distant my end could get was Amy's home office. So I flipped a coin and, ignoring the mantra, decided to troubleshoot the software first. I might as well have flipped a coin that said "idiot" on one side and "moron" on the other.

For someone who is not a professional software engineer, software maintenance is like pulling on the loose strings in a sweater. You just can't resist, but you soon end up with a pile of yarn at your feet. The software infrastructure I had built over a year and a half was soon in strings all around me, and the kitchen lights kept flashing.

So I flipped my coin again, and decided the problem had to be power line interference. Off on another wild goose chase I went, unplugging things all over the house to see if the lights in the kitchen would stop flashing. No luck. By this time I was desperate enough to try the first thing that I should've tried—I replaced the switch that was causing the problem. Magically, the kitchen light stopped flashing, but unfortunately the kitchen light was now the only one in the house that was still working.

Home automation hobbyists use an acronym to describe the maturity of their systems: WAF. It stands for "wife acceptance factor," and it's a measure of just how much nonsense your spouse is willing to put up with before she throws a shoe. Amy was the soul of restraint for the entire time that I was working on this little project of mine, because when it works it's actually pretty cool. I only occasionally heard her walking around the house muttering, "...can't turn a damned light on in this entire place, and I need a keyboard to flush the toilet. Wish he'd just go back to work..."

The Home Automation Incident used up a large portion of Amy's goodwill. She made it known that SHE HAD HAD ENOUGH, that the lights needed to work reliably, and that there was no need, ever again, for the house to speak to her. I think I've got it fixed now; just one more little tweak...

After I was diagnosed, things periodically fell apart in other ways, and not just with my home automation system. I had "long, dark nights of the soul," and occasionally wallowed in self-pity. Parkinson's disease is a movement disorder, but movement problems are only one part of the physical and mental problems it brings. Depression is also a very common symptom of PD. It's a result of the neurotransmitter malfunction that characterizes the disease, and is different than being sad or having a bad day. For PWPs, clinical depression can erode quality of life as much as any of the motor symptoms, and it can be life threatening.

PWPs are at risk for other psychological problems as well, including anxiety, panic, bursts of anger and aggression, paranoia, and delusions. Parkinson's apathy is not as well known, but is just as disruptive, and I began noticing it in myself as I lived with the disease.

Parkinson's apathy isn't depression—it's an inability to start activities or projects, to maintain motivation, and to finish actions, accompanied by a pervasive feeling that nothing matters. I began to have trouble returning phone calls, sending e-mails, attending meetings and volunteer activities, exercising, and having a social life. Every action was exhausting, including making the bed, washing the dishes, or doing a load of laundry. At the end of the day I would often find tasks that I had started but never finished. I felt like I was wading in molasses; every thought and movement was an effort, and it all seemed pointless. I could be cajoled into motion, but I would coast to a stop.

An inescapable sense of numb hopelessness began to invade my thoughts. I often had to force myself to stay active and connected, and I still do. Some days I win, and some days I have to resolve to try again tomorrow.

Apathy is as common as depression for a PWP, but it doesn't get as much notice. It contributes to our tendency to become socially isolated—it looks like disinterest in maintaining contact, and coupled with other communication and speech problems and lack of facial expression, it can make a PWP a "hard interface." It also contributes to frustration and conflict with family members and caregivers since it can look like laziness or a lack of willingness to help. The understanding that it's just another part of the disease isn't much comfort to anyone.

The physical and mental impacts of PD continued to plague me. It was abundantly clear to me how dependent I was on PD medications, and now on DBS. If either were to disappear, my life would become very difficult. I also had a growing recognition that my condition was not going to get better. None of the treatments and therapies had the slightest impact on the underlying disease; at best, they masked the symptoms. I knew that a positive attitude could be a weapon against the disease, but I also knew that no matter how positive I remained, I wasn't going to win against PD. What was the use?

These thoughts and feelings may have been the result of the flawed electrochemical interaction of neurotransmitter chemicals and the billions of neurons in my brain, but it felt to me like my soul crying out for answers and a reason to hope.

I ignored obligations and responsibilities and neglected relationships while, as Amy's grandmother once phrased it, "I sat and stewed on my stool of do-nothing." And I asked, "Why?"

Why me? Why this? Why now? What had I done? I asked the air, not expecting an answer and sure that there wasn't one. I wanted to hold someone or something accountable. And, as usual, all I heard was my own voice. It hadn't occurred to me yet that if I was going to ask, perhaps I should listen for an answer.

MICE, MEN AND MORTALITY

I had always looked forward to the Christmas holidays. When I was young, the anticipation and excitement were almost too much to bear, and my brother and I would "practice for Christmas morning" to ease the tension. "Practicing" entailed getting into bed fully clothed each afternoon leading up to Christmas Day, pretending to be asleep, and then whispering to each other, "Do you think it's time to get up yet?"

We would draw out the suspense for as long as possible, and then jump out of bed and race each other to the Christmas tree in the living room. He always won; he claimed it's because he was older and more agile, but I still think it was because he cheated and wasn't shy about tripping me.

As an adult, I began to look forward to Christmas as a welcome respite from the demands of work life, a chance to spend time with my family, and in later years, an opportunity to try new ways of celebrating the holidays, like food poisoning while scuba diving in Cozumel and broken bones while skiing in Park City. I even looked forward to going back to work after the holidays were over; the "fresh start" newness to old tasks and responsibilities made even the most difficult jobs more bearable.

The Christmas after I retired was the first time in nearly thirty years that I didn't go back to work afterward. The holidays felt like watching the movie "The Return Of The King," the concluding episode of the Lord of the Rings trilogy—an enjoyable experience, but every time you think it's reached the end, it hasn't. Over, and over, and over…

I thought that a perpetual vacation would be a relief; during the most stressful, difficult years of my work life, I fantasized about never having to work again. When it became a reality, it made me uncomfortable. Although I had hopes that one day I'd be able to retire early, I wanted to hit the finish line at full speed, leaning forward and "dipping for the tape" as I once did running the 220-yard dash. John Steinbeck had it right about best-laid plans, though, even if he stole the idea from my distant kinsman Robert Burns (or from Psalm 33, depending on who you ask).

I still counted myself fortunate, though. Unexpected disability is one of the leading causes of mortgage foreclosure and bankruptcy. Parkinson's is also notorious for contributing to relationship problems, fractured families, and divorce. Amy and I had certainly weathered a few storms and had our fair share of water slopping over the transom, but we were still seaworthy. Also, Amy, in true Texas frontier-woman style, had learned to shoot. She said it was to be able to protect me in the future if she needed to; it's possible that she only wanted to keep me polite and humble. It worked.

One of the best decisions we made as a couple was to find a financial advisor we trusted, and to listen to her. She advised us, at a time in our lives when we were absolutely sure we were invincible, to hope for the best but plan for the worst and buy long-term care and long-term disability insurance policies. Her advice could not have been more on target, even though I chafed at the idea of spending money for such a thing when I was obviously so healthy. Having taken her advice will keep my Parkinson's diagnosis from causing financial catastrophe for our family. Although our lives are now radically different, disability insurance will keep us from near-term financial ruin, and long-term care insurance will prevent my eventual need for professional care from bankrupting Amy when the time comes. Things could be much worse—this time, Burns and Steinbeck were wrong.

I was still finding new ways that PD intruded on my life, like the disruption of my sense of smell. Typically, a PWP's ability to sense odors, and consequently the ability to taste more than just the basics, fades away. Loss of the ability to smell can be one of the first symptoms of the disease. In my case, however, my sense of smell went temporarily insane for several months not long after my initial diagnosis, after having been largely absent for many years. For six months, I constantly smelled a pervasive, horrible odor that I could not escape. I even imagined the odor when I was asleep, a combination of rotting fish and burning plastic. The phantom smell was bad enough to make me actively sick to my stomach several times a day.

We tried everything we could to mask or eliminate the smell: chewing gum, breath mints, air fresheners, candles, and unscented laundry soap. Nothing worked. I can advise, however, that if your spouse ever suggests that you put peppermint essential oil in your nostrils to combat a foul odor, you should back away with your fingers in your ears. I've only recently stopped sneezing, crying, and smelling peppermint-scented burning plastic and rotting fish.

PD can also cause digestive system slowness and difficulty swallowing. The resulting combination of severe heartburn and choking when eating and drinking can be disconcerting and dangerous, and for more than a year I slept sitting up in a chair to keep from waking up choking. A combination of medications and diet changes eventually let me sleep in a bed again, but sleep often eluded me for other reasons.

On one occasion, after a dinner that didn't settle well, I again lay awake all night. Even my wonder drug for gastric reflux was ineffective, and the heartburn burned through. At about 5:30 AM, I thought I felt well enough to try to sleep. After only a few minutes of dozing, though, I woke up choking. It had happened before, but this time was different. I was coughing and wheezing, but also unable to catch my breath. Amy tried to help me to relax and calm down, but I was caught in a vicious cycle. Stress makes all Parkinson's symptoms worse, and not breathing is stressful. In this case, the stress triggered a bout of dyskinesia. Again I found myself getting a week's work of exercise in just a few minutes, but this time while not breathing.

After claiming several times that I really was getting better, and a short battle with my mother-in-law (Amy didn't get her fortitude by accident), I arrived at the emergency room where they did doctor stuff and determined that I was coughing and not breathing well. After x-rays, an EKG, chest listening and thumping, and a couple of hours of calm breathing, the episode passed and they let me go home, with stern warnings not to fail to breathe regularly or there would be consequences.

For a brief, irrational time, I thought I might die. It was an odd realization for someone who's lived half a century and once considered himself to be indestructible, but my mortality slapped me in the face. It's one of those unpleasant, "mustn't touch it" topics, but PD is life limiting. Asphyxiation from choking, aspiration pneumonia, acute injuries and complications from falling, dementia, and depression can all reduce life expectancy. Ultimately, life itself is life limiting, and PD symptoms are treatable with exercise, medication, and surgery. The fact remains, though, that there is not yet a treatment that significantly changes the rate of progression or course of the disease.

I understood that no one knows when his or her own end will come, and that each of us could be hit by a bus or a falling safe at any moment. However, the likelihood is that I won't have a Wile E. Coyote experience, but that I'll live out my days with Parkinson's and probably die from it. That realization made me impatient with foolishness, meanness, stupidity, and cruelty, and with bad choices and bad judgment, especially my own. We all have so little time, and we waste so much of it.

Realizing, at long last, that I was not immortal moved me to reconsider important philosophical questions. I was an analytical thinker, and answers and reasons were important to me, but these were some of the most critical questions in human existence. Why am I here? What do I do next? How do I keep going? I had made an informal career of asking questions such as these, as if there was something virtuous in asking. There is a difference between asking questions and seeking answers, though, and I was beginning to see that asking without really seeking was a waste of time. I realized that my lack of faith in a transcendent reality was the safe, fence-sitting approach. If I didn't commit to anything that couldn't be rigorously justified, I was less likely to be wrong, embarrassed, ridiculed, hurt, or shamed. Sadly, I was also less likely to see the fullness and richness of life with a higher purpose.

Discovering I had an incurable, degenerative disease brought "meaning of life" questions into sharp focus, and I began to realize that I was unsatisfied with my conclusions, and with the basic, non-rational beliefs on which I had built them. But, I had no idea what to do about it, and I had never had a sense of being guided by a spiritual force or a sense of revelation. I prayed, but all I heard were my own thoughts and the sound of my own breathing. I felt trite and foolish, and like I was grasping at straws, abandoning my rationality as soon as things got tough.

I also began to fear that PD was having effects on my judgment and decision-making ability. How could I know what was real and what was fantasy? Can the cognitively challenged have real faith, or as some have said, is all faith a form of mental illness?

Near despair, I gave up trying to figure it out. To my surprise, that turned out to be the right answer.

DISOBEDIENCE

Before I learned I had Parkinson's, I was a scuba diver. I loved everything about diving: the sense of community and camaraderie among people with a common passion, the technical and scientific character of the knowledge required to do it well, the complexity and variety of the equipment, and the freedom I felt while I was diving. Whether I was in the gin-clear, eighty-two-degree water of Cozumel with 300 feet of visibility, or in the forty-five-degree blackness and near-zero visibility at the bottom of a Texas lake, I felt at home. Even in my frequent vivid dreams of flying, I was wearing scuba gear.

I probably didn't have to stop as soon as I did, but I was safety-minded and conservative. I didn't want to hurt a dive buddy or a student in the classes I helped to teach, and I didn't relish the thought of drowning because my PD symptoms suddenly reappeared at just the wrong time. I searched for something to replace diving, and I mourned the loss.

Through a complex series of circumstances and events, I began pistol shooting. Although it's a counterintuitive sport for someone with Parkinson's to adopt, it's surprisingly similar in unexpected ways to scuba diving. There is a community of like-minded enthusiasts who share knowledge and help each other. It can be dangerous, but with caution, training, and experience, the danger is controllable and manageable. It requires a specialized body of knowledge, but is accessible to almost anyone willing to put in the time and effort to learn. And the equipment, for a gadget geek and someone with an engineering mindset, is endlessly interesting. There's always something new to learn and discover.

About a year after I began shooting in small, local competitions, I found myself on a plane with my Aggie friend Gene on one side and a very large man and his fiancée on the other. We were all on the way to Las Vegas, them to get married, and Gene and I to head out into the Nevada desert for a four-day defensive handgun-training course. We planned to learn defensive handgun safety, gun handling, and marksmanship techniques, but we agreed we would be satisfied if we merely avoid shooting the wrong

WALKING THE CROOKED PATH

things, including each other.

It's actually not quite that bad. Although I experience many of the major motor and non-motor symptoms of PD during the course of a typical week, they don't usually happen at the same time, and I'm able to squeeze off a shot or two during the lulls. And, I have the luxury of unloading and putting the gun down if I'm shaking, stiff, or clumsy; it doesn't generally come upon me without warning. There's always plenty of time to shout, "Hit the deck!" and toss the gun away like a hand grenade.

We had planned the trip for several months. We collaborated and argued about firearms, accessories, ammunition, and range time. We spent innumerable hours discussing the merits of John Moses Browning's masterpiece (the Model 1911 .45 ACP semi-automatic pistol), the pros and cons of pistols made from Tupperware, and the meaning of life and our place in it. And now we were leaving the civilized world behind, on our way to the badlands to learn to shoot with proper adult supervision.

My large seatmate, who was now wearing a panicked look and beginning to sweat as we approached Vegas and his impending wedding, was growing larger by the minute. He was already getting premium value from his ticket price by taking half of my seat as well, and was busy trying to acquire the other half. I discovered something new, however; Parkinson's dyskinesia could be an excellent defensive tool. The more he encroached, the more I thrashed. I considered making noises, but thought that might be over the top.

I enjoyed telling people I was a shooting enthusiast—I liked their tolerantly amused expression until they realized I was serious, followed by their intense desire to know exactly where and when my next shooting excursion would be. I had advised them to avoid Nevada for the next five days.

When I was first diagnosed, I was tempted to decide out of hand that there were some things I shouldn't do. There are, of course: teaching scuba classes, tightrope walking, diamond cutting, and being a tattoo artist come to mind. But there are other things, like shooting, that I can do, with a sober, realistic approach, the right preparation, and the willingness to wait for the right time. PD is a thief, and I don't want to let it take things that I can still hold onto for a while. I had begun by "fighting back," but I was beginning to believe that was the wrong metaphor. Perhaps the right approach was less direct confrontation and more civil disobedience. PD may have power, but I could still refuse to allow it free rein. PD wanted me to sit at home—NO, I'm going to go shooting in Nevada with my friend. PD wanted me to sleep all day—NO, I'm going to the high school to talk about computers with smart, eager young people. PD wanted me to resign to my fate and give up hope—NO, I'm going to hold on and find new reasons for hope. PD wanted me to stop exercising and sit in front of the computer—well, okay, but I'll do better next week. No philosophy is perfect.

During my week in Nevada, my way to question PD's authority over my life was to learn to clear a room and shoot from cover. It's not likely I would ever need to use those skills since being a Navy SEAL numbered among the things I probably shouldn't do, but if needed, I would be ready. And, I loved thumbing my nose at Parkinson's.

We arrived in the southern Nevada desert after a leisurely dinner on the outskirts of Las Vegas and a pleasant moonlit drive. As we settled into our hotel room and ran a few errands around town to gather supplies for the week, we discovered that there is no path between two points in the entire town that doesn't pass either through a casino or past a fireworks stand. I had been to Vegas on business a number of times over the years, so I expected the slot machines at the airport and in the grocery store. The roulette table in our hotel room was a surprise, though.

We rose early the first morning, packed guns, holsters, accessories, sunscreen, bottled water, Gatorade, and food into our rental car, and headed twenty miles across the desert to our 6:30 AM check-in at the training facility. As the sun rose over the mountains, we were greeted by our first glimpse of the landscape where we would spend the next four days.

"I thought we were in Nevada. How did we get to the far side of the moon?" said Gene.

"Oh, it's not that bad," I replied. "Look, there's a dead cow—you'd never see that on the moon. At least it's nice and cool—only sixty-five degrees. It probably won't get much hotter than that." Stupidity often sounds like optimism.

We arrived at the facility slightly before the appointed time and waited briefly in a line of other students for the staff to open the gates. At the exact moment the clock hit 6:30 AM, we entered the facility after being greeted warmly at the gate. This was our first exposure to both the precision and professionalism we would experience throughout the week.

As directed, we headed to the sign-in area to check in for our class and have our guns and holsters checked for safety. Since they didn't yet know about my steel-trap mind, the sign-in staff thought it best to write the number of my assigned range on my hand with a Sharpie—1A. They then verified that our guns were neither too small nor too large, our ammunition would probably not detonate prematurely or with unexpected fanfare, our holsters covered our triggers, we weren't smuggling concrete or peanut butter in the barrels of our pistols, and we were otherwise prepared to be instructed. We then headed to the classroom to receive our official welcome and to sign paperwork saying that, regardless of what happened in the next four days, no matter who was at fault, irrespective of which body parts were affected, and with no consideration of intent, true culpability, or gross negligence, we were solely at fault now and for all time. I signed without reading. If there's a war in the Mideast now, I think I agreed, it's my fault.

We then headed to Range 1A, where we met our range master and his team for the first time. They were all dressed alike: crisp short-sleeved gray uniform shirts, bloused black fatigue pants, boots, and baseball caps. Sharp, professional, and squared away, they were also each friendly, approachable and genuinely welcoming.

At this point, I spoke privately with the range master and explained to him that I had Parkinson's disease, but that I could usually tell when I was having problems that would impact my ability to participate. He nodded his understanding and said, "Safety is a very important part of this course, but we'll keep an eye on you as we do for everyone, and you just take things at your own pace." My remaining concerns faded into the background.

We spent the day going over the basics: the Four Rules of Firearm Safety, the rules of the range and the facility, range commands, chamber checking and magazine checking, and other safety-related subjects. We actually didn't fire the first live round until the afternoon, which was fortunate—I learned that I had been doing almost everything wrong, and I had a significant amount of unlearning and bad-habit breaking to do.

The day ended with a lecture on the moral and ethical issues associated with deadly force, and I was once again struck by the thoughtfulness and serious deliberation that had gone into this course. These were not gun nuts gleefully popping off rounds in the desert—they were instead professionals with a deep understanding of the awesome responsibility inherent in choosing to use firearms for self-protection and sport, and a recognition that this is a controversial subject even among well-intentioned, intelligent people. Thoroughly exhausted, we headed back to town for an evening of pistol cleaning and rest.

We spent the second day practicing and learning to draw correctly from a holster, and to reholster without shooting ourselves. Among many other things, we also learned the value of dry practice and the Three Secrets of Handgun Marksmanship. I had thought there was only one secret—shoot enough rounds and eventually you'll hit the target. Again, I was wrong.

We learned quickly. My new vocabulary now includes timeless nuggets such as "tap, rack, flip," "chamber check and mag check," tactical reload," and the popular "finger straight, look and move, check, lock, strip, rack rack rack, insert, rack, point in." It's not what it might sound like.

PD decided to reassert itself on the third day of class. I had hoped but didn't really expect to avoid a "bad day" during the week, and I awoke with the familiar, stiff, slow, shaky feeling and clumsy, shuffling gait that greets every morning. As occasionally happens, though, my morning handful of pills only brought nausea and disorientation, and no relief. I knew I wasn't safe to handle a gun, so I went to class and just watched that morning. I began to feel better by the afternoon, but my bad day brought me up short.

Who was I fooling? What was I doing here? I had PD—I wasn't going to recover, and I would never be any better at shooting or anything else than I was at that moment. Why bother? Why waste my time? I really just needed to get on the plane, go home, sell the guns, and get realistic. Feeling low and discouraged, I talked with Gene, who was also exhausted and dealing with his own challenges. Together we decided to stick it out for one more day, the last day.

I awoke on the last day dreading a repeat of the prior day's challenges, but thankfully, both Gene and I felt much better. PD is capricious and unpredictable, but that unpredictability cuts both ways. We arrived at the facility and spent the morning practicing and preparing for the final test scheduled for that afternoon. After we had practiced for several hours, though, the range master gathered us together and told us he had a surprise.

"We're going to have a competition this morning. You'll be competing against each other in a single elimination, man-on-man tournament that simulates one of the threat scenarios we've discussed—a multiple adversary hostage situation." Oh boy, I thought. As they used to say in Strategic Air Command, here was an "opportunity to excel." I resolved to try to apply what I had learned and make the best of the situation.

The scenario involved three targets made of differently colored steel armor plating. Competitors competed in pairs; each competitor had their own set of three targets that they were required to shoot in the proper order, while in direct competition on the same range. The first target was a gray man-shaped steel silhouette placed fifteen yards from the firing line, with a small white-painted steel square mounted on an axle next to the head of the silhouette, which would flip away when struck. The gray silhouette represented the hostage, and the small white square represented a hostage-taker standing behind the hostage with only a portion of his head showing. The two other targets, placed at twenty-five yards and painted blue and red, represented two other adversaries. The goal of the competition was to first shoot the white square and flip it away without striking the hostage, and then to shoot the blue target and the red target in that order, before your opponent did the same thing. Whoever finished first without hitting the hostage won the round. If both competitors hit the hostage, both were eliminated. If it sounds easy, try it in 100-degree heat wearing a concealment vest and presenting from a concealed holster.

The competition proceeded, with some shooters doing well and some less well. Gene raised the bar when he stepped up to the line and hit all three targets in order with three well-placed shots, well before his opponent, to the cheers of the class.

My turn finally came—I was part of the last pair in the first round. We stepped up to the line and I tried desperately to remember what to do as I heard, "Shooters! Firing drill. Load, chamber check, mag check, and return to the holster." My training kicked in and I didn't even think as my hands automatically moved through the drill we'd been taught over the last three and a half days. I heard, "Ready, fire!" and I smoothly (for me) swept my vest to the side, presented my 1911 .45 ACP from the holster, pointed in at the first target while snapping off the thumb safety, established the right sight picture as I removed the slack from the trigger, focused on the front sight, pressed the trigger to a surprise break, and trapped the trigger as I heard a "ping" and saw a blurry image of the white target slap back. Without consciously thinking about it, I moved the sights to the blue target, reset the trigger, and repeated the process, and again with the red target. I heard the instructor say, "when you're satisfied with the condition of your weapon, return to the holster," so I executed a tactical reload and reholstered. It was only then that I discovered that I had won the round. I was so shocked I nearly soiled myself.

As luck would have it, I was paired with Gene for the second round. In a repeat of the first round, we both fired three shots and both connected three times for a perfect round. His red target fell about a tenth of a second before mine did, though—he eliminated me from the competition, and although I would have loved to have beaten him (he's an Aggie, after al), I was as thrilled for him as I would have been for myself. After a bye and another perfect round, he won the competition and received the Man-On-Man Competition Challenge Coin. If I had to lose, that was the way to do it.

We both went on to take the final test and finish the course—neither of us was the highest scorer, but we weren't the lowest, either. We both had areas for improvement, but we were both safer and better shooters. And I answered or reaffirmed some of the questions I asked myself on the third day: Why bother? Because although I can fail, I cannot fail to try. Why waste my time? It isn't a waste—it is a refusal to curl up and die. Who am I fooling? No one, including myself. I have PD, and I don't expect it to just go away.

I hope for a cure, but I don't anticipate one in my lifetime. However, my willingness to be disobedient to PD can't depend on the hope for a cure. I continue to work as I can to help find one, but I also get up every day with the hope of learning something new, of meeting and overcoming challenges large and small, and of trying to go just a little farther every day than I think I can.

I struggled to come to terms with Parkinson's disease and to live without surrender, but that was not the most important struggle before me. The radical disruption PD brought to my life stripped me of the carefully crafted defenses I had built, and showed me how vulnerable I was. I believed I had control of my life; my sense of control was an illusion. I believed I had all the answers; I was asking the wrong questions. I believed that I could hide from the big questions and ignore the voids in my life behind a wall of reason and rationality; I still felt something important was missing. And I believed that the wrongs that had been committed against me gave me leeway to silence the still, small voice that I pretended not to hear inside me.

God, Whom I had ignored, denied, derided, disproved, hidden from, argued against, and rationalized away, would not be silenced. He found me, and quietly showed me I was wrong.

REVELATION

Gene grimaced as I asked my question. I had noticed that he often did, and I wondered if he knew it. I suspected that I had begun to tax his patience. We were talking about the Bible (the book of Hebrews, to be exact), and it was making both of our heads hurt.

"I'm not getting how Jesus could have been both fully divine and fully human," I said. "Some sort of quantum state, like Schroedinger's cat, maybe?"

When Gene returned home from Africa, we resumed the discussions about faith that we had begun by email. I reiterated that I was unashamedly without belief, and Gene reiterated that he was unashamedly of deep belief. For a time, it appeared that we were simply incompatible on the subject. Gene even told me, "You're not my project; you're my friend. If you don't believe what I do, so be it. We can still talk about other things and we can still shoot." That was fine with me, too, but we still continued to talk, and I continued to ask questions.

I talked with him about both my academic and emotional objections to religious faith, and he listened without arguing. I ran down my list of "unanswerable questions," discussed passages from the Bible and pointed out the logical and factual errors, talked about religious scholars and philosophers I had read, and expounded about Russell's Teapot, Pascal's Wager, invisible pink unicorns, blind watchmakers, irreducible complexity, tornadoes and 747s, monkeys and typewriters, and other arcane subjects. Gene listened, and admitted at one point that, although he had been a missionary for many years, he had never heard some of the things I talked about. He didn't refute any of them, but instead continued to tell me about his experiences. After a particularly taxing conversation on one afternoon, he asked me, "If you're so sure you're right, why are you still asking questions?"

His question brought me up short. I had described myself to believers for years, and to Gene when we first met, as a "failed seeker." As I considered his question, it occurred to me that I used the description to both distance myself and to claim kinship. I wanted to believe, but I also wanted someone else to do the hard work. I wanted to be convinced, but only by someone who could first pass my test. If they could, I wouldn't have to take the risk of being wrong and, more to the point, of being disappointed yet again.

I went to visit Larry, the friend who had originally asked me how PD had influenced my theology, and who then had paid for it by reading the hundreds of closely spaced, tightly reasoned pages of my answer. He spent the weekend with me, and he had arranged a dinner with a group of guys he had met that he thought I would like. They were similar in a few ways; they all lived in the same city, they all had two legs, and they all professed faith in God. The similarities ended there, though—they talked, argued, disagreed vehemently, agreed more vehemently, called each other names, got mad, got glad, and thoroughly enjoyed each other's company. And no two of them believed exactly the same things. I heard as many views as there were people in the room, ranging from what I recognized as fundamentalist to surprisingly liberal viewpoints. I was astounded, and encouraged.

One of the guys asked me if I could describe why I didn't believe in God. I started down the laundry list, and began to recite the manifesto from memory. He listened patiently for a while, and then stopped me gently.

"No, I didn't ask what the reasons for not believing in God are. I asked why YOU don't believe in God. What are YOUR reasons?"

I started to protest that those were my reasons, but then I stopped. It was a fair question. I had spent years gathering other people's arguments as ammunition to defend my unbelief. Stripped of those things, what were my reasons?

Slowly, I stammered, "I've never felt like He was there. I've asked for His help, and he hasn't given it to me. I've prayed, and He hasn't answered. I don't feel anything."

The guys around the table nodded, and one spoke up. "Me, either. I've never had the experience of God's presence."

I said, "How can you commit your life to something you don't even know is real?"

"It's not about feeling; it's not as if you put your faith coin in the machine and you get your happy feelings in exchange. It's about choice—I choose to believe. It made sense to me after I'd chosen, but the fact that it makes sense didn't make me choose."

Later, discussing the evening with Larry, he agreed. He also thought I was trying too hard to force God to fit into my box. He suggested that God might have plans of His own, and maybe I should see what they were instead of dictating them.

I was thoroughly confused and despondent. I had spent my whole life figuring things out and controlling outcomes and events with knowledge. It was all I knew how to do. I was never going to think my way to God, and I was never going to get there any other way. I gave up, again, for what I thought would be the last time.

I went home and continued to visit with Gene. I loved him and his family, and I treasured my time with him. For six months or more, I visited him once a week and we would shoot, go for walks, go to lunch, talk, and enjoy each other's company. We also studied the Bible and talked about faith.

I figured it could do no harm. I wasn't seeking any longer; I had given up. I continued to read and study with him; it was interesting, and the stories illustrated principles I could agree with. I began to read on my own, and I found still more to agree with. The inconsistencies and flaws that I perceived were still there, but as I read and studied, they began to take on less importance.

Amy had taught a confirmation class at our church when our children were young, and she had shared some of the content with me. There were several kinds of truth in the Bible, she said. She talked about six kinds of truth: moral, historical, scientific, symbolic, proverbial, and religious. I remembered our conversation, and when I encountered one of my Biblical "sticking points," I tried looking at it from the perspective of another kind of truth, instead of coming to a full stop.

I kept asking questions during my weekly visits with Gene. Slowly, without fanfare, blasts of trumpets, or fireworks, I realized that I had stopped asking to show how smart I was, and that I was asking to seek answers. The transition was slow and almost imperceptible, but I had reached a tipping point. I still had doubts, uncertainties, and questions, but I was looking at them from a different perspective. I didn't know when, how, where, or why it had happened, and I couldn't explain it, but it was true.

I believed.

RESOLUTION

Recently, a good friend died. His death was completely unexpected; he left behind a large and loving family, and literally thousands whose lives he had enriched. He was a man of deep faith in God, and he lived his principles wherever he went, not like a coat he could take off when it was inconvenient, but deep in his bones, an inseparable part of who he was.

He always seemed to have a new spin or an interesting view, and he had a remarkable ability to get deeply involved in the details and then suddenly step back and look at the big picture. He didn't let the minutia bog him down—he just kept going and arrived at the solution when others couldn't even see the path.

His faith in God was as much a part of him as his big feet and booming voice. It came from his family first, from many generations back, but as an engineer and successful businessman, he was never one to accept a conclusion without examining the logic. I did the same thing, but we had different backgrounds and experiences, and I came to a different conclusion. I was focused on examining the notes and couldn't hear the music all around me. I'm starting to hear the music now.

I believe. After a lifetime of asking questions, not to get the answers but to show there were none, I believe. After repeatedly proving to myself and to others that God couldn't exist, and even if He did He didn't care, I believe. Even though I can't explain it and it's not rational, I believe. Even though I'm afraid that people important to me will not understand and will worry that PD is taking over my rational mind, I believe. After fighting it, wishing I could, and giving up countless times for almost forty years, I believe. I'm a little late to the party, but I believe.

I'm still working out the details, but the music is there. It's faint at times, but I hear it. I may never be able to play in the symphony, but I finally hear the music.

I haven't given up my respect and regard for critical thought and scientific inquiry. I don't suddenly reject thousands of years of steady social and scientific progress, nor do I deny that there is beauty in rational discovery and, as the physicist and Nobel laureate Richard Feynman put it, "finding things out." There's no need to.

I have instead broadened my world with a recognition that the God I rejected, but who never rejected me, speaks with many voices, uses many tools, and is a master of many kinds of truth. My world is not diminished; instead, it is bigger than I imagined, and the missing pieces are starting to fit together. I'll always be a questioner and seeker of deeper truth; I have that freedom. But, the minutiae don't bother me as much anymore. I don't care how many angels can dance on the head of a pin.

Why do I believe? Because it feels right and because I choose to. I didn't arrive here through rational analysis, but through a wholly personal experience that I can describe, but not explain. I can't provide a methodology for coming to faith, or for falling away, for that matter. All I can say is, "This is what happened to me."

What do I believe? That's a harder question. I have a sense that almost all of us, even the devout and learned believers, will eventually find that we had most everything wrong. When Paul told the Corinthians, "For now we see through a glass, darkly; but then face to face. Now I know in part; but then shall I know even as also I am known," I think he knew of our tendency for misinterpretation and error. However, when I consider the multiple voices, the many tools and methods, and the varied ways of expressing Truth that God can employ, I am surprised to find that a very old creed that I first learned long ago but that I still remember expresses the core of what I believe:

I believe in God, the Father Almighty, maker of heaven and earth;
And in Jesus Christ his only Son, our Lord;
Who was conceived by the Holy Spirit, born of the Virgin Mary,
suffered under Pontius Pilate,
was crucified, dead, and buried;
The third day he rose from the dead;
He ascended into heaven, and sits at the right hand of God the Father Almighty;
From thence he shall come to judge the quick and the dead.
I believe in the Holy Spirit, the holy catholic church, the communion of saints, the
forgiveness of sins, the resurrection of the body, and the life everlasting.

There is much here open to interpretation, disagreement, ridicule, or rejection. I know that better than most—I did all those things. Nevertheless, the essence of my belief lies here, in The Apostle's Creed.

My journey is not over—the most recent segment has barely begun. I recently learned that the Veterans Administration has decided that incidents during my period of service in the Air Force are the likely cause of my PD, and they have determined that my disability is service-related and that I am unemployable. That's not what Amy and I hoped for when we set out from Austin on a journey now in its twenty-ninth year, but according to one great philosopher, "you can't always get what you want."

My struggle with Parkinson's disease will not be easy, and I know there may be times when I question my newfound faith and rage at the God who has given me so much. I can only hope and pray for wisdom and strength if that time comes. I know God can take it, though—He's taken much worse from me.

I don't know why I have PD; I don't believe it's a punishment or a test, but I do believe there may be a purpose. In any case, there is no one to blame or to direct my anger toward. I don't know why my father did the things that he did, and I don't know why God allowed it to happen. The only person who carries responsibility has been gone for almost fifteen years. What my father did to me was inexcusable but not unforgivable, and I have forgiven him; not for his sake, but for mine. He was not simply an evil man who caused me pain and anguish. He walked his own crooked path, and probably dealt with pain and anguish of his own that I know nothing about. I'm still angry at him for what he did, and for the harm it's caused me and my family, but I'm no longer tormented by it.

There is always the possibility that Parkinson's disease will be cured tomorrow, next week, or next year, but I choose to live my life exuberantly and with purpose whether that happens or not. I choose to disobey PD's control over my life. I choose to love my family and friends openly and unselfconsciously, and to continue to learn, grow and stretch for as long as I can. And I choose to make God central in my life, in spite of doubts, uncertainties, and unanswered questions.

I choose to believe.

###

55182913R00062

Made in the USA
Charleston, SC
22 April 2016